Self Confidence

for Women

How to Build Self-Esteem, Overcome
Social Anxiety, And Empower
Your Life for Success!
A Guide to Stop Self-Doubt and
Gain Confidence.

Jennifer Campbell

—

2

original author of this work can be in any fashion deemed liable for any hardship or damages that may befall them after undertaking information described herein.

Additionally, the information in the following pages is intended only for informational purposes and should thus be thought of as universal. As befitting its nature, it is presented without assurance regarding its prolonged validity or interim quality. Trademarks that are mentioned are done without written consent and can in no way be considered an endorsement from the trademark holder.

Table of Contents

—

7

Introduction

Everyone desires to be confident, yet very few have been able to develop it in all facets of their life. A lack of self-confidence can ultimately become the most significant hindrance to finding happiness, success, and fulfillment.

Unfortunately, too many people often are unable to see the effects low self-confidence has on their lives, blaming their failures on outside factors instead. They blame a tough dating scene for not finding the right partner.

They are desperate to find a better job but don't know where to start because the job market is so competitive. They wish they could follow their dreams but can't afford to fail. On the surface, these kinds of excuses seem like they are legitimate outside barriers, keeping us from finding true happiness. However, when further examined, the justifications are all rooted in a lack of self-confidence. Past experiences have helped to develop your current mindset, and the past unknowingly plagues us as we grow into adults.

As adults, we often waste a ton of energy attempting to appear confident rather than developing real confidence. The importance society puts on outside appearances only reinforces the pressure to show false confidence.

This is just intensified with the popularity of reality television and social media. It has become the norm for our society to appear one way to everyone else, rather than focusing on making the changes internally that will allow us to alter our sense of self.

For example, many people will post photoshopped images to their social media profiles in the hope of garnering a ton of likes to help increase their shaky self-esteem. Hence, the façade of confidence trumps genuine, unwavering confidence. So, many people are afraid to admit they lack confidence because it is seen as a personal weakness, while others wish they could have more confidence, but don't know where to start.

If you suffer from a lack of confidence, it will continue to hold you back, even if you become adept at faking it. The great news is, you can be one of the few people that learn how to build an undeniable, persistent, and genuine level of self-confidence that won't be affected by outside circumstances.

This guide will provide you with tips and strategies to develop confidence in all areas of your life. You will also learn the ways you can develop a strong sense of self and unconditional self-love to get you through any challenges that you might face in your life.

The only difference between those who are successful and those who fail in life is the willingness to keep trying. Having confidence will provide you with the drive and the ability to work toward your goals without your limiting beliefs standing in your way.

Chapter 1

Self-Esteem and Confidence

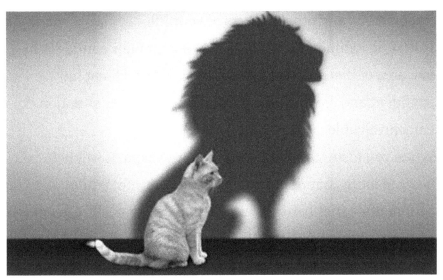

Self-esteem and confidence are often used interchangeably to describe an individual's level of assurance, poise, self-respect, and security. While these two concepts are often related, they are not the same.

The main difference is that self-esteem is a constant, while confidence is something that fluctuates. It is vital that you are able to foster a strong sense of both. To do this, you must first understand the origins of both and how each can be affected and changed.

Confidence vs. Self Esteem

Confidence is a huge part of your overall well-being. Being confident will help with your career, relationships, self-image, interactions, and other aspects of your life.

It isn't uncommon for someone to be extremely confident in one area of their life, yet insecure in another. Being fully confident and comfortable with yourself in every situation is truly invaluable.

When you foster a strong sense of self-esteem, it will help you become more confident in all areas of your life. While confidence varies between circumstances, your self-esteem is a continuous part of your self-concept.

The higher your self-esteem, the more likely you will be comfortable facing a variety of situations in your life. Self-esteem is an underlying trait that directly affects how you perceive yourself in all circumstances. Self-esteem can be tricky because a lack of self-esteem will manifest in a variety of ways.

Generalized self-doubt is one way that low self-esteem can manifest. If you have low self-esteem, you may automatically assume that you won't be good at a task and will either give up or subconsciously sabotage yourself into failing. This is your self-concept trying to prove why it has low self-esteem.

If you repeatedly fail in a variety of circumstances, your subconscious says, "I told you this would happen." During every situation that you face, negative self-talk will rear its ugly head, telling you that you will fail, you'll look stupid, you'll embarrass yourself, and those others will harshly judge you. This negative self-talk is not accurate, but instead, it originates from low self-esteem.

Humans are social creatures, which gives us the ability to pick up on indicators of high or low self-esteem. It is these indicators that often affect how we respond to one another. Those who have high self-esteem are more likely to get a job, create social connections, strike up conversations, etc.

It isn't that most people are looking to hurt those with low self-esteem intentionally, it is just a natural tendency for us to be attracted to those who exhibit confidence. We are all self-serving beings, innately trying to get ahead and when someone exudes confidence, it indicates they can help us get ahead in life.

The way in which we present ourselves can be a clear indication to those around us of our levels of confidence and self-esteem.

Physical cues like slouching, talking sheepishly, or a constant downcast gaze, all indicate low self-esteem.

During conversations, expressing doubt, frequent verbalization for a need for reassurance, or indecisiveness, are also clear signs of low self-esteem. It is relatively easy to see these kinds of signs in young children and teenagers; however, many adults have learned to hide their insecurities.

Many of us have all adopted the fake-it-until-you-make-it attitude.

Unfortunately, we are so focused on faking it that we never work toward fixing the underlying issues.

Another way in which low self-esteem manifests itself is a confidence-contingent outlook. It displays itself when a person relies entirely on their accomplishments to feed their self-esteem. This is far harder to spot in ourselves and other people.

This kind of low self-esteem makes us have the need to succeed at everything so that we can feel good about ourselves. They may also feel the urge to put others down to feel superior, which feeds their confidence temporarily. The critical factor in these cases is always contingent on outside factors and is always temporary.

It results in the continuing need to feed the self-esteem monster in an attempt to escape your true feelings. It is a vicious and draining cycle that is incompatible with peace, happiness, and real self-esteem.

If you know how to build your confidence in any situation, it will help you to develop your overall self-esteem. Confidence in separate situations is a necessary building block to retrain your mind to think more confidently.

As your confidence becomes more natural, self-esteem grows and becomes a part of your self-concept.

Thus, developing unwavering self-esteem, as well as knowing how to build confidence in specific situations effectively, are both essential components for success and well-being. So, how do you know if you lack confidence and have low self-esteem?

5 signs to determine if you have low self-confidence

Here are 5 signs to determine if you need to work on your self-esteem and confidence.

1. Constant Indecisiveness

Being indecisive often is a sign that you don't trust yourself to make the right decision. Doubt and insecurities accompany this.

Those who lack self-esteem are frequently riddled with self-doubt. Being indecisive in many situations may indicate low self-esteem, while having it in one or two situations may show a lack of confidence in those particular situations.

For example, if you are a new business owner, you may spend more time making decisions than a seasoned entrepreneur because you are frequently second-guessing yourself. As you learn and develop the appropriate skills, you'll increase your confidence. Thus, knowledge and experience will improve confidence in individual situations.

2. Focused on Outside Reassurance

Self-esteem comes from your self-assurance, which means that you are confident in all situations and aren't swayed by the opinions of others. One symptom of low self-esteem is often

---

the frequent fluctuation in your mood based on the actions of others.

Again, if this only happens in a few situations, it merely indicates that you may have a lack of confidence in those areas. However, if it is a reoccurring theme across the board, it is an indication that you have low self-esteem.

For example, if you always need to be told that you look nice to feel good about your appearance, you likely have low confidence about your self-image. If you also need constant reassurance at work, in relationships, and during social interactions, this likely indicates that you have low self-esteem.

3. Hesitant to Speak Up

Being reluctant to voice your opinions is another sign you might have low self-esteem and lack confidence. It indicates an underlying doubt in what you have to say. It might mean that you are unsure if your opinion is valid, or you tell yourself that others are uninterested in what you have to say. You might fear that by speaking up, it will cause others to dislike you.

Having low confidence in a particular area may cause you to be hesitant about voicing your opinion because you may fear you are not knowledgeable enough in the field. If you are a new business owner and attend a networking event, you may not feel confident to share your thoughts with a 20-year veteran.

If you continuously fear speaking up, it is an indication that you are suffering from generalized low self-esteem. This might cause negative thoughts of doubt that ultimately prevent you from speaking up.

4. Inability to Take Criticism

Being focused on outside reassurances and a failure to take criticism often coincide in individuals with low self-esteem. When you need others' approval to feel good, then hearing criticism can be crushing. For these individuals, criticism is always taken as a personal attack on the ego rather than being looked at as feedback.

When you suffer from low self-esteem, the opinions of others are valued higher than your own self-worth, the criticism is taken as truth, instead of mere opinion. When you have high self-esteem, you use these criticisms as helpful feedback and are able to listen and discard it as an untrue opinion.

5. Give Up Easily

Self-doubt is a substantial cause and symptom of low self-esteem. Nobody is an expert when they try something for the first time, and it requires perseverance and overcoming obstacles before you can succeed at anything. Someone with wavering esteem can become easily defeated when they fail the first time.

While your confidence may feel shaky when you are first embarking on a new endeavor, with the appropriate level of self-esteem, you will be able to figure out how you can increase your confidence.

When you have low self-esteem, the shaky confidence can become overwhelming, causing you to give up, protecting yourself from the potential consequences and discomfort that may come with failure.

Chapter 2

How Limiting Beliefs Can Affect Your Self-Esteem

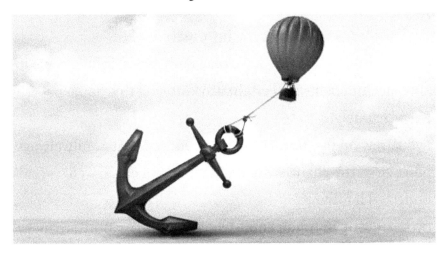

Many people suffer from low self-esteem because of their limiting beliefs. Limiting beliefs are blind and unhealthy beliefs that stop and constrain you from achieving success in your life.

They are self-imposed prison walls that you have built to protect yourself from the fear of failure and humiliation. It is a fake label that you give yourself to lock yourself in a cocoon of safety.

The fear of stepping out of your comfort zone is so intense that you give up at the first hurdle that you come too. They ultimately stop you from going after your dreams. Our beliefs come from two sources, our experiences, and our influences.

Our Influences

From an early age, we are bombarded with opinions and information from our family, society, and the people closest to us. As we grow and form bonds with our classmates and others, our conscious and subconscious minds continue to absorb, filter, and process the information.

All of the interactions we have on a daily basis, influence us to think, act and believe a certain way. Most of this happens subconsciously.

If you grew up in a household that believed that family always comes first, the chances are that you have a close, well-connected family.

If you grew up around people who think the wealthy are lucky and get all the breaks, chances are you believe that your ability to become wealthy is a steep, and impossible climb. If you grew up in a family that believes in a good education, chances are you believe the same and now expect your kids to get a good education as well.

Our Experiences

We learn from every experience we encounter in life. Whether you consciously learn from the experience or not, doesn't matter. Regardless, our minds tend to form beliefs based on single, significant experiences or cumulative experiences of the same nature.

In fact, many of our limiting beliefs are a result of our experiences. As a kid, if you performed poorly on a science test, you may begin to believe that science is a subject that you will never understand or succeed at.

If you've repeatedly been cheated on in your relationships, you may think that there are no good people in the world and that you'll never find love. If you've been passed up for a promotion at work, you may believe that you are unqualified to perform at a higher level.

Both our influences and our experiences work to determine what our beliefs are, and usually form during our childhood. As you begin to understand where your opinions come from, you can start to question them and ultimately change them.

How Limiting Beliefs Keep You from Living Your Life

Throughout your life, you've constructed beliefs in yourself and about the world, which can directly contribute to your way of life. What's surprising is that these beliefs can also have a physical effect on you.

The more reinforced the idea is, the more impact it can have on your body. Whether you know it or not, your body shows the physical and mental manifestation of limiting beliefs that surround your self-image.

Your limiting beliefs will cause you to feel like you will never be able to achieve a goal. This can result in decreasing your self-confidence, ultimately losing your self-esteem in the process.

As your self-esteem falters, you might start avoiding trying new things and going on new adventures because you will believe that the risks and dangers surrounding the experience to be destructive and even fatal.

This will result in you complaining to others and placing blame, without discovering the underlining source of trouble. This can result in you starting to lose the balance you want in life that is necessary to keep it healthy and running.

Limiting beliefs, tend to cause self-judgment that is unhealthy, leading you to feel the need to put up a mask and hide your true self from the world. The fear of not accepting who you are could result in you losing your self-identity without even realizing it.

The limiting beliefs that you hold can result in physical changes to the body as well. This includes continuous and persistent agitation, depression, anxiety, indecision, bad temper, queasiness, and other emotional problems.

This can change who you are and the way you talk to others. The tone of your speech changes and you will tend to be negative. It can cause you to always find ways to complain and blame others for your problems and failures.

Identifying Limiting Beliefs

The first step to overcoming your limiting beliefs is to identify them. Living with your limiting beliefs can lead you to live a mediocre life, one that is significantly different from your potential.

Unfortunately, limiting beliefs can be challenging to identify. Before you can begin to identify your limiting beliefs, you need to learn to keep track of your self-talk and become aware of the judgments that your subconscious is making.

By knowing how to keep track of the way you talk to yourself, you will be able to identify the limiting beliefs that run through your mind during conversations. Getting rid of the bias of your subconscious mind is another vital step in finding your limiting beliefs.

Some of the most common limiting beliefs include:

- I can't be my real, authentic self because I'll be judged.
- I can't fall in love because I'll get my heartbroken.
- I can't ask for what I want because I'll get rejected.
- I can't trust people because they will eventually betray my trust.
- I can't pursue my dreams because I will most likely fail.
- I don't need to be successful, so I'm not going to even strive for success.
- It's too late to pursue my dreams.
- I'm nothing special because I've never accomplished anything exceptional.
- I don't deserve happiness because I'm not good enough.
- I hate the way I look, and there is nothing I can do to change.
- I am too weak and will never be able to find the strength to change.

Chapter 3

Overcoming Your Limiting Beliefs

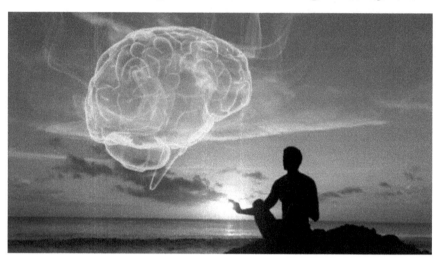

Now that you have identified your limiting beliefs, it is time to work on overcoming them. Unfortunately, most people don't take the steps necessary to do this because they believe that by having an awareness of their limiting beliefs, they will be able to think differently about their circumstances and lives.

While being aware of your limiting beliefs will encourage you to think about them differently, a significant number of your limiting beliefs have a ton of emotional investment behind them, which is ultimately where the problem lies.

Whenever you have a tremendous level of emotion invested in something, it can create a barrier to change. In order to make lasting change, you have to cut your ties. In fact, the deeper the conviction or belief, the more difficult you'll find the process and the longer it will take.

Lying at the cornerstone of any change that you want to make is the willingness to adapt to the changing conditions and circumstances that surround you. This is especially true when it comes to changing your limiting beliefs.

Choose the Outcome You Desire

The very first step that you have to take to overcome your limiting beliefs is to choose the outcome that you desire. When you choose your desired outcome, you are able to gain more clarity about what it is in your life that you would like to change.

You have to ask yourself some tough questions and thoroughly consider your answers. You need to ask yourself:

- What goals would I like to achieve?
- What's currently preventing me from achieving my goals?
- What kind of person would I ideally like to become?
- What specifically do I want to change?
- What specific beliefs aren't working for me?
- What limiting beliefs are preventing me from achieving my desired outcomes?

Once you have become clear about the limiting beliefs that are holding you back, you can start the process of overcoming these limiting beliefs and increasing your self-esteem.

Questioning Your Limiting Beliefs

It is important to remember that your limiting beliefs are only as strong as those references that support them. Often, the limiting beliefs that you hold have a plethora of references that have helped to influence and shift your perspective on reality. It is important to remember that these references started out as ideas, which turned into opinions, which later became your beliefs. If you want to change your limiting beliefs, you have to change your perspective and opinion about them. You can start to throw doubt on your limiting beliefs by asking yourself:

- Is the belief accurate?
- Have I always believed this? Why?
- Was there a time that I didn't believe this? Why?
- Is there evidence that can disprove this limiting belief?
- Are there times when this belief doesn't make rational sense?
- Will this belief help me get what I want? Will it help me reach my goals?
- What is the exact opposite way of thinking about this belief? How is this helpful?

These questions are designed to help you increase perspective and the possibilities of your situation. They are meant to encourage you to think outside the box, so you can begin to shift how you think about your limiting beliefs.

Consider the Consequences of Your Limiting Beliefs

Now that you have begun to throw some doubt on your limiting beliefs, it's time for you to consider the possible consequences of holding onto your limiting beliefs. To do this, you need to think long and hard about the following questions.

- What will the consequences be if I'm not able to make this change and eliminate this limiting belief?
- How will not making a change affect me emotionally? Physically? Financially? Spiritually? In my relationships?
- How will not making a change affect my life?
- Are there short-term consequences of not changing my life? What are they?
- Are there long-term consequences?
- What makes making this change now so essential?

The more pain that is associated with holding onto your limiting beliefs, the higher the motivation you'll have to make positive changes in your life. That's why it is essential to move through each of these questions, one at a time to fully experience the pain. You want to feel the anger, think about the regrets, experience the guilt, and allow yourself to cry.

Choose a New Empowering Belief

In order to move forward after you've considered the consequences of holding onto your limiting beliefs, you need to choose a new empowering belief. It is vital that you make sure that this new belief is believable. If it isn't one that is believable, the chances are high that you will be unable to condition your psyche.

To unlock your new empowering belief, you need to consider the goal that you want to achieve, the person that you want to become, and the core values that you want to maintain. Once you have considered these, you need to ask yourself the following questions from a third person's perspective:

- What would this person likely believe while pursuing this goal?
- What would this person believe about themselves?
- What would this person believe about their goal?
- What's their attitude like? How do they think about the goal?
- How would they think about the obstacles they encounter along the journey?

Now, you need to take some time to consider the advantages of this new empowering belief and how it can improve your life and your circumstances. Ask yourself the following:

- What benefits can I expect from using this new belief?
- How will it help me reach my goals?
- How will it change my life for the better?
- How will it help in both the long-term and short-term?
- How will this new belief make me feel about myself?
- How will this new belief empower me moving forward?
- Why is this important?

The more reasons that you can find, the higher your motivation will be to break your old patterns of behavior and replace them with a new, empowering belief system.

Condition your New Belief

Now that you've committed yourself to change your limiting beliefs to new empowering ones, the next step is to begin to condition your new beliefs into your psyche progressively. One way to do this is through the process of visualization. Spend time every day visualizing yourself, in your imagination, using your new way of thinking in your day-to-day activities. Take particular note of the actions you take, the decisions you are making, how you talk to others, and how you talk to yourself.

Think about your newly formed attitude and how your new beliefs are going to help you manifest the life you want. You are in essence imagining a new you in your minds-eye. Another process that you can use is the process of anchoring this new belief to condition it into your nervous system. This involves anchoring a sensation that is physical to your body that will allow it to automatically enable you to get into an optimal state of mind that corresponds to your new empowering belief.

It's not easy to overcome your limiting beliefs, but with a significant amount of work, introspection, and time, you'll be able to overcome the limiting beliefs that have been holding you back and build your self-confidence.

In the next chapters, we will look in more detail at the limiting beliefs that usually afflict people with low self-confidence and how to remove them using appropriate strategies.

Chapter 4

5 Steps to Building A Rock Solid Self-Confidence

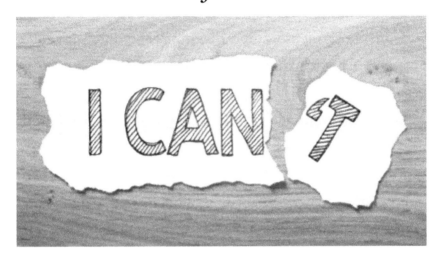

Building self-confidence is an ongoing process that needs determination and energy. Here are some steps to think about when you are trying to build yours:

Step 1: Step Out Of Your Comfort Zone

If you are going to have unshakeable confidence, you have to be willing to step out of your comfort zone so that you can do things out of the ordinary. You have to stir up that urge burning within you to be extraordinary.

Perhaps you have a brilliant idea that your belief could benefit your company, but you do not know how to share that with your boss. Perhaps you have a crush that you never dared to approach.

The problem that comes with not acting on these desires is that you will stagnate right where you are. Truth is, when you fail to explore new experiences, you are letting fear take away your sunshine. You are simply digging deeper into your zone of comfort. The hole that you have been sitting in for several decades now.

Yes, it may be intimidating to make the first approach into the unknown, risking being embarrassed by failures. But if you think about it, it's just 'FEAR' – False Evidence Appearing Real. What is the worst that could happen? Often times, you are just overthinking. Stepping out of your comfort zone can be so daunting, but it is important if you wish to fulfill your life's purpose and have unshakeable confidence. This could be the way you can finally prove to yourself that you can achieve anything you set your mind to.

After all, what is the worst that can happen? You can share with your boss and steer the company to success, or the boss simply turns it down. You could ask that girl or boy out, and they could say either yes or no – You also get your answer without wasting too much time guessing. Either way, it is a win-win situation.

The secret to having solid confidence starts with you!

One thing that I will tell you for sure is that to get out of your comfort zone; you have to start by setting micro-goals that will all eventually add up to the bigger picture. Micro-goals simply refers to small pieces of the larger goal you have. When you break your bigger goals into chunks, accomplishing them becomes quite easy, and you will have so much fun while you're at it. This will also build up your momentum to keep pushing until you have reached your target.

So, we suppose that you have a business idea or strategy that you would like to share with your boss but haven't gotten the courage to do it. What you can do instead is break your major outcome into smaller goals that eventually yield similar outcomes. Take small steps to get started, no matter how small it is. Instead of taking the big leap and feeling overwhelmed, starting small will take the pressure off you. When you do this, you simply make things quite easy to digest and make follow-ups easy.

So you like that girl or boy and have no courage to tell them how. But he or she may not be single in the first place. So your micro goal should be to establish a rapport with them first before you dive into the deepest end of things. Even before you ask them out on a date, get to know who they are by just initiating a short conversation with her/him. Isn't that better? This does not sound like you are stalking them.

That said, you have to appreciate that when you set micro-goals, it allows you to step out of your comfort zone. As you achieve your micro-goals one after the other, you will realize that every small win can help you get the confidence you need to move forward. Challenge yourself that you are going to do something out of the ordinary every day and see how that grows your confidence.

Step 2: Know Your Worth

Did you know that people with rock solid confidence are often very decisive? One thing that is pretty admirable with successful people is that they do not take too much time trying to make small decisions. They simply do not overanalyze things. The reason why they can make fast decisions is that they already know their big picture, the ultimate outcome. But how can you define what you want?

The very first step is for you to define your values. According to Tony Robbins, an author, there are two major distinct values; end values and means values. These two types of values are linked to the emotional state you desire; happiness, sense of security, and fulfillment among others.

Means Values

These simply refer to ways in which you can trigger the emotion you desire. A very good example is money, which often serves as a mean, not an end. It is one thing that will offer you financial freedom, something that you want and hence is a means value.

Ends Values

This refers to emotions that you are looking for, like love, happiness, and a sense of security. They are simply the things that your means values offer. For instance, the money will give you security and financial stability.

In other words, the means value is the things that you think you desire for you to finally get the end values. The most important thing is for you to have clarity on what you value so that you can make informed decisions much faster. This, in turn, will give you a strong sense of identity, and that is where you draw everlasting confidence from. You have to be in control of your life and not the other way around.

One way you can do that is ensuring that you define your end values. You can start by dedicating at least an hour or two each week to write down what your end values are. To get there, start by stating what your values are that you'd like to hone to get to your dream life.

Some of the questions that might help you put things into perspective include;

- What are some of the things that matter most in your life?
- Are there things that you do not care about in your life?
- If you were to make a tough decision, what are some of the values that you will stand by and what are those that you will disregard?
- If you have or had kids, what are some of the values you will instill in them?

Step 3: Create your own happiness

Happiness is a choice, and also the best obstacles are self-generated constraints like thinking that you're unworthy of happiness.

If you do not feel worthy of joy, then you also don't believe you deserve the good things in life, the things that make you happy and that'll be precisely what keeps you from being happy.

You can be happier. It is dependent upon your selection of what you focus on. Thus, choose happiness.

Happiness is not something happens to you. It is a choice, but it takes effort. Don't wait for somebody else to make you happy because that may be an eternal wait. No external person or circumstance can make you happy.

Happiness is an inside emotion. External circumstances are responsible for just 10 percent of your happiness. The other 90% is how you behave in the face of those conditions and which attitude you adopt. The scientific recipe for happiness is external conditions 10%, genes 50 percent and intentional activities - that is where the learning and the exercises come in - 40%. Some people are born happier than others, but if you're born unhappier and practice the exercises, you will end up happier than somebody who had been born more joyful and does not do them. What both equations have in common is that the minimal influence of outside conditions on our happiness.

We usually assume that our situation has a much greater impact on our happiness. The interesting thing is that happiness is often found when you quit searching for it. Enjoy each and every moment. Expect miracles and opportunities at each corner, and sooner or later you will run into them. Whatever you focus on, you may see more of. Pick to concentrate on opportunities, decide to focus on the good, and choose to focus on happiness. Make your own happiness.

Step 4: Be Ready to Embrace Change

Have you ever found yourself obsessing about the future or the past? This is something that many of us find ourselves doing. However, here is the thing; the person you were five years ago or will be five years from now is very different from who you are right now.

You will notice that five years ago, your taste, interests, and friends were different from what they are today and chances are that they will be different five years from now. The point is, it is critical that you embrace who you are today and know that you are an active evolution.

According to research conducted by Carol Dweck, it is clear that children do well at school once they adopt a growth mindset. In fact, with the growth mindset, they believe that they can do well in a certain subject. This is quite the opposite of what children with a fixed mindset experience because they believe that what they are and all that they have is permanent.

Therefore, having the notion that you cannot grow only limits your confidence.

What you should do to embrace all that you are is stopping self-judgment. Most of the time, we are out their judging people by what they say, how they say it, what they wear, and their actions. In the same way, we judge ourselves in our heads comparing our past and present self.

For you to develop a strong sense of confidence, it is important that you start by beating the habit of self-judgment and negative criticism. Yes, this is something that can be difficult at first, but when you start to practice it, you realize how retrogressive that was.

You can start by choosing at least one or two days every week when you avoid making any judgment at all. If you have got nothing good to say, don't say it. If there is a negative thought that crosses your mind, you replace it with a positive one. Gradually, your mind will start priming to a state of nonjudgment, and it will soon become your natural state of mind. This will not only help you embrace others but also accept yourself for who you truly are.

Step 5: Be Present

Sounds simple, right? It is important and necessary that you build your confidence. By being present, you are simply allowing your mind, body, and soul to be engaged in the task at hand.

Let us imagine speaking to someone that is not listening to what you are saying. This is something that has probably happened to a good number of us. How did you feel? On the other hand, imagine speaking to someone, and you feel like you were the only person in the room. Feels pretty special, huh?

The reason why you feel special is that they were present at that moment. They paid very close attention to what you were saying, feeling every emotion with you. They were engaged in the conversation at a deeper level. This way, you can retain information while still experiencing empathy.

To be present, you have to develop a mental double-check. This simply means that you should mentally check-in on yourself regularly. To do that, you have to develop a mental trigger or calendar when you ask yourself where your mind is. This is the time when you act as an observer of your mind. Are you thinking of dinner reservations while in a meeting? Do you think that you are not good enough? To call yourself out of these negative thoughts means that you mentally check in on yourself every often. Once you have the answer to your question, take in a deep breath and bring back your focus on your most important things.

Chapter 5

Daily Habits to Consolidate and Increase Your Self Esteem

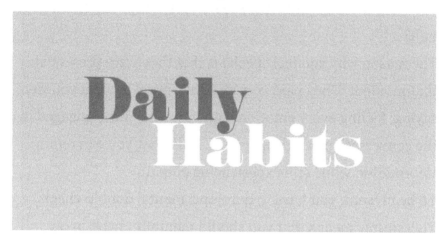

Now that you've have discovered how to identify and overcome your limiting beliefs, you can begin to rebuild your self-confidence by boosting your self-esteem. To do this, you have first to change your self-perception.

You need to change how you look at yourself and how you view yourself. Everybody has self-perception. Everyone has a mental picture in their minds of who they are, what they are capable of, and where they are going.

If you suffer from low self-confidence, you have a negative view of these things. You probably feel that you are not worth much of anything and that whatever you try will result in mediocrity or failure.

You have to work on your self-perception if you want to increase your self-esteem and build your self-confidence. To start the process of improving your self-esteem, you need to incorporate these daily habits into your life.

Forgive yourself

If there is any shortcut to healthy self-esteem, this is probably it. When you manage to forgive yourself, you take your self-esteem to another level. It's all about kindness to ourselves and having compassion - not only for others but for ourselves. (Do not confuse this with self-pity, which is toxic.)

One reason for low self-esteem is because we feel guilty for something we've done or left undone, so it is crucial to forgive yourself. As soon as you've completed this, your self-esteem increases, and you will also be capable of forgiving others.

Be forgiving to yourself, accept your mistakes and vow to never repeat them, forgive yourself for your flaws (you're only human and do not have to be perfect) and work on your own strengths. Forgive yourself for your sins and do not repeat them if possible.

The changes you'll see when you figure out how to forgive yourself are absolutely remarkable! Occasionally disorders go away; occasionally self-forgiveness clears the previous energy block to allow wealth to come into your life. Just do it and see what forgiveness is going to do for you in your lifetime.

Grow Your Knowledge

Another step to growing your confidence is ensuring that you gain knowledge both in your personal and professional endeavors. There is always that area that you feel you are limited in knowledge and understanding.

If you want to have more confidence, then you have to demonstrate mastery in this area. You can expand your knowledge by taking online courses, attending similar conferences and events, as well as reading books. The other thing that you can enjoy while gaining knowledge is tele classes where you get to interact and engage in discussions with your peers. This will go a long way in improving your level of confidence.

Change Your Self-Talk

Self-talk is merely the act of talking to yourself, either mentally or aloud. It is any thought that pops into your head in reaction to external stimuli. The way that you feel about situations depends on what you tell yourself.

If you think about the situation negatively, it will lead to negative emotions like irritation or anxiety. Thinking about the situation positively will lead to positive feelings like excitement or happiness.

When you are working on increasing your self-esteem, you become more aware of the constant self-talk that leads to negative feelings, and you can replace it with positive self-talk that encourages higher levels of self-esteem.

For example, if you are always telling yourself that you are fat every time you look in the mirror, you need to stop and replace these thoughts with words of encouragement.

In this example, you have trained yourself to look at areas of your body that make you insecure and reinforce your insecurity by saying "I'm fat."

If you teach yourself to look in the mirror and appreciate your body or focus on an area that you feel good about, over time, this will shift your self-image and confidence.

Practice Affirmations

Affirmations are simple, positive statements that you say about yourself to change negative thinking patterns. You can say a set of affirmations every day or use them to replace negative self-talk.

Affirmations help to improve self-esteem by implanting new beliefs to replace beliefs that cause low self-esteem.

When you are trying to change your automatic thoughts and negative self-talk, it is helpful to have a set of affirmations to use in place of the old, negative thinking patterns that you have developed. With enough repetition, affirmations will become implanted into your subconscious mind.

Soon we will talk in more detail about positive affirmations and how they can support you in developing a solid self-confidence.

Stop Comparisons

You have to recognize you are unique. You also have to realize that you never get the full story and that everyone puts on a front in an attempt to disguise their insecurities.

When you compare yourself to others, you are merely comparing yourself to the façade others are presenting to the world.

Everyone has thoughts, doubts, insecurities, judgments and other inner battles that they deal with within their minds.

You also need to stop using comparisons to make yourself feel good about yourself. It is tempting to do in an effort to feed your own ego, but it turns into a vicious cycle.

When you use comparisons to make yourself feel better, your brain will automatically use it to make you feel worse. The only way to escape this is to cut yourself off from making comparisons between yourself and others.

Eliminate Judgment

Judgment is one of the most destructive and least productive habits you can develop. Unfortunately, few live a life that is free form judgmental thoughts. Judgment and true confidence are incompatible. One can never experience genuine peace while holding onto judgments.

Judgment becomes habitual in us; we naturally do it without even realizing it. We judge ourselves as a form of punishment for not being perfect, and we judge others in an attempt to make ourselves feel better.

People who are truly happy with themselves do not feel the urge to judge others or themselves.

The first step on the path to this kind of freedom is accepting that there is nothing perfect in the universe.

You need to learn to take yourself as you are and accept others in the same way. Everyone came into this world with different personalities, have had various experiences that have shaped us and we all continue to face challenges. Judging anyone is unfair.

Give up guilt

Guilt is one of the most destructive emotions, and the world is filled with guilt-ridden men and women. The worst is that it is an unnecessary feeling. An entire book could be written about the uselessness of the emotion. It wouldn't be an issue if we could feel guilty for a few moments and then go on with our lives, but sadly, lots of people live with chronic guilt.

Why do we always feel guilty? Because we have been conditioned to feel guilty our entire life. Consciously or unconsciously, since our youth, our loved ones, friends, society, school and religion have fed our remorse and enforced it through the punishment and reward system.

As kids, everybody reminded us constantly of our poor behavior and compared us to other kids which were behaving so much better. Guilt was used to control us.

The bad thing is that this sort of treatment leads us to feel guilty, even if we did not do anything bad. Also, for quite a very long time, guilt was related to caring. If you really care you need to feel guilty, and if you do not care and do not feel guilty, you're a terrible person. Nothing is farther off reality. Guilt does not serve you at all; it just causes you real psychological harm and causes you to feel despicable. Stop the guilt illusion today. There's a massive difference between feeling guilty and learning from your mistakes. Guilt always brings punishment, which comes in several forms including depression, feelings of inadequacy, deficiency of self-confidence, inadequate self-esteem, and the inability to appreciate others and ourselves.

The fantastic thing is that the more you work on your own self-esteem along with your authenticity and being around the right people the less guilty you will feel. At any time you feel guilty, remind yourself that it's an unnecessary emotion, and learn from the error. That's all you've got to do.

Focus on your strengths

If you often around toxic people, they may be tempted to call out your flaws. Ignore them. While it's good to know about our flaws - we understand them, we do not need anyone always reminding us it's better for us to become aware and focus on our strengths.

- What are the top five personal qualities and professional strengths?
- What do you do best than others?
- What are your most important personal and professional achievements?
- What makes you unique and strong?

Then it is time to fortify them. Practice them and concentrate on them - the ones you've got and the ones you want.

Learn to say NO

There could be persons in your own life who will attempt to convince you to do things even if you don't want to do them, and occasionally because we wish to please everybody, we say "YES" to them even if our inner voice say "NO." Saying yes when we'd like to say "NO" harms our self-esteem and after we can feel sort of sad or angry.

Learning how to say no will enhance your life a good deal. You will get more of YOU because every time you say YES when you mean NO you get rid of a little bit of yourself and your self-esteem go down.

When you decide that a "Yes" is a "Yes" and a "No" is a "No", you will feel better. This implies fewer obligations and although telling your friends and family "NO" is hard at the start, the benefits are great.

The most successful people say "No" quite often. So, be certain to say "NO" without feeling guilty.

Surround Yourself with Positivity

While it isn't a great move to blame our failings on others, often other people can be responsible for our low self-esteem. This is true if we hang out with the wrong crowd – if our friends are prone to pointing out our flaws instead of building us up and raving about us.

And this is why you need to avoid toxic people. Ironically, if you consider everything that we have said in the first chapter, it is often the people who lack confidence who feel the need to try and damage ours. They make us feel small to make themselves feel bigger.

If you know negative and toxic people like this, then you should make a conscious attempt to not hang out with those kinds of people anymore. Likewise, you should spend more time with the positive people who love you.

And if you do have to spend time with people who are damaging your esteem? Then just consider their motives for everything they say. If they are criticizing you, then is it because they genuinely think you've done something wrong?

Or is it because they are jealous? Or because they're just a negative kind of person? Don't let it affect how you feel about yourself.

Improve Yourself

Many of us have things that we don't like about ourselves. But often, those things can be improved. And the sheer act of trying to improve can often be enough to give us a tremendous boost in self-worth.

So, if you don't like the way you look, then consider the ways you can improve your style perhaps to look better. If you feel too 'skinny' then bulk up. If you feel overweight, then lose weight. If you think you are a little slow-witted, then work on your repartee. If your math lets you down, go get lessons!

Incorporate Self-Care

Neglecting your own needs can contribute to low self-esteem, as well as being a symptom of low self-esteem. Self-care is merely doing something because it makes you happy.

It can be as simple as relaxing in a bubble bath, enjoying a massage, or taking a walk by yourself. Self-care is often looked at as selfishness. People often feel guilty for spending time on themselves because they think that it is taking away the happiness of others.

The first step to change this is to recognize you are worthy of time and attention and release any thoughts that cause guilt.

Next, you need to think of one thing that you can add in on a regular basis that is 100 percent for you.

Tell your loved ones that you are doing it and be as committed to yourself as you have been to everyone else.

Let go of Perfectionism

Perfectionism is often a cover-up for insecurity. It is also the number one enemy of confidence. Perfectionism comes from an underlying belief that you must be perfect to deserve love and acceptance from yourself and others.

It indicates that an individual place his or her self-worth on accomplishments and defines his or her self-concept based on actions. This mindset leads to drastic fluctuations in mood and confidence and immense pressure to always get it right.

You need to let go of your perfectionistic tendencies. You have to foster unconditional love and acceptance for yourself and know you are separate from your actions and accomplishments.

The more willing you are to accept yourself when you make mistakes, the higher your self-esteem will become.

Celebrate Daily Victories

It can become overwhelming when we are trying to change any aspect of our lives. Changes take time, and it can only happen with daily actions.

There have been plenty of people who have been able to overcome shyness and develop healthy self-esteem, but it wasn't accomplished overnight. To stay motivated on your path to increasing your self-esteem and building your confidence, you have to recognize and celebrate the small victories.

Celebrating small victories when working toward any goal will also help to build your confidence. You deserve credit and have to be willing to give yourself recognition. If you are always focusing on how far away you are from reaching your end goal, your journey may turn into a struggle, filled with doubt and disappointment.

Instead, celebrate the small accomplishments along the journey and become filled with the encouragement and the energy to continue.

Be Grateful for What You Have

Individuals with low self-esteem tend to focus on the negative experiences and lack in their lives. It is easy to focus on what you want but don't have, and it takes an effort to change this outlook.

Expressing appreciation and gratitude for everything in your life will transform your perspective during each moment and eventually alter your perceptions of yourself and the world. When practicing gratitude, be thankful for the blessings in your life, and who you are as a person. Take a moment to list three unique things that you appreciate in yourself and three things that you are grateful for in your life. Try to incorporate a practice of gratitude for yourself and the world on a daily basis and see the impact it has on your overall self-esteem.

Exercise Passionate Faith

One of the qualities I admire about confident people is that they have faith in a supreme being. They believe that the creator of the universe has a purpose for every living soul. In other words, the reason why we are on earth at this time is to discover and fulfill our higher purpose.

In other words, they seem to have perfect knowledge that when they forge through with the creator's plan, achieving success is just a matter of time. Therefore, if you truly want to achieve success, you must have faith that it is possible. It is important that you have unwavering faith in your potential. When your faith is filled with passion, then there is a high likelihood that you will follow your true purpose.

Set Realistic Expectations

The quickest way to kill your confidence is to set high expectations for yourself. Setting goals and working toward them can help you build your confidence. However, if you set unrealistic standards, you will only end up feeling defeated. If you have something that you want to work toward, come up with a realistic goal that you can work on today. Keep your goals small and attainable and be sure to celebrate each small victory.

Expect to Be Confident

Did you know that expectations are faith in actions? At this point, you have already envisioned yourself being confident and how that would make you feel. When you are confident, you will talk, act, and move assuredly and with so much zeal as you pursue your goals. This is when you know that you have the sight, emotions, and actions of a confident person. In other words, you will be better positioned to achieve above and beyond your expectations. When you expect to be confident, it becomes a reality.

Like we have already said, confidence is not something that happens overnight. You have to constantly put these actionable tips into practice for months. Start by writing down ways you intend to apply these action plans. This way, you know exactly how it would be like to take action towards your goal. When you act on them, you start realizing tremendous improvements in your confidence, and soon this translates to solid confidence, happiness, joy, and ultimate success in life.

Chapter 6

How to identify and overcome Self-Defeating Behavior

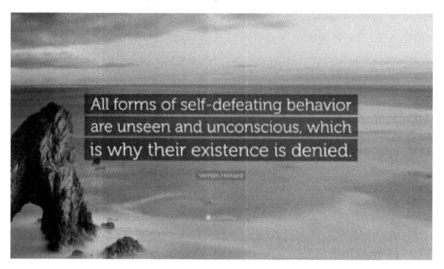

All forms of self-defeating behavior are unseen and unconscious, which is why their existence is denied.

Vernon Howard

Self-Defeating Thoughts. We usually do not realize we have them and yet they're strong enough to dictate our choices. They are strong enough to steer our lives in particular directions, directions which might not be supportive or healthful, directions that might not result in a fulfilling life. And all we see is negative.

Self-defeating ideas are automatic and habitual, marginally below our consciousness. These thoughts tell us we aren't good enough, worthy or deserving of being joyful, causing us to lose our decision to proceed toward our potential.

Overeating and nasty behavior can seriously lower how you feel about yourself. Sometimes that's the point. Traumas throughout your life can make you feel like you don't deserve to be attractive, socially satisfied or financially stable.

You may need professional help to totally turn this attitude around, but there are also some things you can do on your own. We'll see them soon.

In the meantime let's see what are the traits that characterize a self-defeating person.

3 Signs of Self-Defeating Behavior

This unfavorable trait commonly starts in early adulthood and in various circumstances. Individuals who have this type of personality are more inclined to stay away from experiences which he or she will take pleasure from. They rarely or never have lasting or successful relationships with friends, family or even a special someone.

There are also instances wherein the individual exhibiting self-defeating behaviors engage in relationships which he or she will suffer from. If you wish to know if you or someone you know has this type of behavior, you have to identify 3 of the most common signs.

1. If you check the relationships of those who have this behavior, one sure sign is that they will never have any lasting and fruitful one. In most instances, they would rather choose undesirable situations which will only lead to failure, maltreatment and even dissatisfaction. Even if they know that there are other options that have more favorable outcomes, they still chose those which will only lead to sadness and frustration.

2. Individuals who have this behavior reject any chance of being happy. They do not engage in any fulfilling activities even if they have the ability to socialize, meet new friends and have fun in the process. They do not want to be with good people. They constantly reject those who treat them well. When it comes to choosing a partner, they would rather choose one which will provide him or her with an unfulfilling relationship.

3. Individuals who have this type of behavior would never accept any help from other people. However, they provide others with excessive help which were not solicited. Also, individuals with self-defeating behaviors are capable of helping others achieve their goals. However, when it comes to himself, he or she is incapable of achieving whatever is desired or wanted.

These individuals use this kind of behavior to face their everyday life. It prevents them from being happy and successful. As you can see, this having this type of attitude will bring anything good to one's life. It will only become a vicious cycle not unless steps are taken to get rid of it.

Those are signs that you could have SDB. You also have to admit to yourself that you could have a problem because SDB is a problem and one that gets progressively worse. In order to break the cycle of escalation, you need to recognize it as a problem. These are easier said than done but remember that the first step is always to the problem identification.

This is the foundation of the discovery process. Without knowing what the problem is you cannot move forward. Just like any scientific approach to a problem you need to start by defining the problem and proceeding from there.

Understanding the Origin of it All

What are the origins of this behavior? These behaviors do not just spontaneously come into existence. You need to reexamine and take a good look at yourself for you to be able to identify where this particular trait comes from.

Frequently self-defeating thoughts stem from infancy. This is when we create assessments to ensure our security and to protect our loved ones, the very people we depend on for sustenance.

For example, if your parents had been very controlling and almost always made your choices for you, then they took away your ownership of your decisions which meant that you felt that you were not responsible for the consequences of your actions. So what happens? You start blaming other people and as you do this you fall into a pattern of blaming those around you. The origin of which was a problem with your relationship with your parents.

—

What you need to do is think back to the first time you exhibited the SDB and remember the events that you were going through during that time. These questions can help you dig deeper:

- What kind of problems were you experiencing?
- What big event trigged the first time your SDB?
- What really hurt you?
- Which have been your emotions about it?
- What was your reaction to that?

These kinds of questions will help jog back your memory to help you remember the underlying situation during that time. Remember to keep all that information in a journal so that you can easily remember it. You need to identify the problem and try to remember what your situation was during that time. This will help you determine and understand if any of those had any impact on the unfavorable trait that you currently have.

Sometimes people misjudge the origin because they expect it to stem from a super traumatic incident in their life. However, it is quite possible that the origins can be quite mundane. It means that you need to carefully plot the history of your self-defeating behavior. As an example, it could be that the source of your SDB was a rejection from a woman way back in junior high. This is because not all people are the same, some people are more sensitive than others and some people take rejection differently from others. Very often, the resolution of the problem is achieved by understanding which needs have remained unsatisfied.

9 Ways for Breaking the Cycle of Self-Defeating Behavior

The standard of our thoughts impacts not only how we act and interact with the world, but the way we see ourselves, and ultimately, what we believe we're effective at. This is why it is so important to recognize and work on, self-defeating thoughts, or deeply held values and ideas that are inherently limiting.

It's one thing to realize that you're having a self-defeating thought. Most people are aware enough to recognize when they're in a negative thought pattern. But the hard part is changing it. Here are 9 tips to help you get started.

1. Know What Triggers You

The first step is to identify these thoughts. Often self-injurious thoughts can include the words "always" or "never". As an example: *"I will never recover"*, *"I can never concentrate"*, *"I can never get the job done"*, *"I'm always the least attractive"*, *"I'm always worse than others"*, etc...

Another way to recognize these thoughts is to ask yourself: "How do I feel, emotionally and physically, while feeling this thought? Is this thought giving me energy or is it taking it off? "If you are feeling being limited, then self-criticism is futile rather than constructive self-reflection.

As soon as you've identified the self-injuring thoughts that you have, focus on if you live them. This can help you understand what situations and individuals trigger them.

2. Create a shortlist

Write down your self-damaging thoughts on a piece of paper, this will surely help you sort out what emotion lies behind some of your harmful behaviors.

List at least ten feelings. Good examples are feelings of rejection, manipulation, embarrassment and even getting hurt physically or emotionally. These are far better than writing general ones such as anger.

3. Write What You Think

Right after creating a shortlist, you need to write down the things that you commonly think of every time feelings such as these are triggered. This time, you can be as general as possible. For example, if you feel rejected, you can write a general statement related to what you may be thinking such as nobody cares about you and that you will never find someone who you can rely on.

4. Pay Close Attention to Your Thoughts

After listing all the thoughts associated with each trigger feeling, the next step is to focus on these thoughts. Try to think of pleasurable situations and think about how you felt during that day. That situation which you are going to think about must be the direct opposite of one thought related to one trigger feeling. This will help you realize that if you are in a good mood and state of mind, you will be seeing this in a different way.

5. Replace" I cannot" with "I won't."

When you're feeling especially self-conscious, it's easy to begin believing that you cannot do something, when in reality, it is truer that you probably just do not want to, because it has the potential to make you super uncomfortable. Replace "I cannot" ideas with "I won't." Do not let your anxiety eclipse your own ability.

6. Replace "I Must" vs. "I Can"

So often we take our lives for granted, failing to bear in mind that what we have today is what we once only imagined. An excellent way to remind yourself of this is to replace the term "I must" with "I can". Rather than: "I must finish this project," believe: "I can finish this project."

7. Bear in mind that you're spotlighting yourself.

Nobody is thinking about you with as much frequency, scrutiny and focus as you are. Nobody. How can we know that? Because all of them are too busy spotlighting themselves. Nobody is focusing on your life how you're, nor are they judging, nit-picking or making assumptions about you the way you do on your head.

8. Quit confusing honesty for truth.

You may honestly feel something, but it doesn't mean it's the truth. Honesty is transparency, it means expressing just what you're experiencing and perceiving. Truth differs, it is objective. Understanding the difference is a must.

9. Seek some help

Getting rid of this kind of behavior is never easy and it cannot be done overnight. Thinking of good things whenever you feel bad will help. Aside from that, it will also be a lot better if you have a support person who can help you go through the entire process of getting rid of this kind of behavior.

Start looking for a safe, supportive and kind person - a friend, a mentor, a mental health professional or a clergy person - to help you determine the wrong beliefs you're bringing without even realizing it.

Next time you feel yourself getting bogged down by your unwanted thoughts or self-defeating behavior, follow these easy strategies to navigate out of routine each time. And remember: you do not need to be your ideas, habits or attitudes. You're not your behavior. You always possess the capability to change your mindset to navigate yourself out of hardship.

Mindfulness can supply you with the tools you will need to reprogram your conditioning, it requires some work, but the benefits are priceless.

Lastly, you can engage in physical and fun-filled activities. This will help you realize that there's more to life than being alone, sad, frustrated and other negative feelings.

Chapter 7

Meditation for Building self-confidence

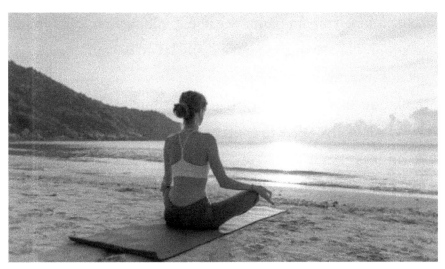

Another incredible tool for enhancing your confidence is meditation.

Many people are reluctant to give meditation a chance, thinking of it as being somehow mystical or associating it only with Eastern religion and philosophy. This is not what meditation is in reality at all.

Instead, meditation is simply the act of concentration – of consciously choosing how you want to direct your attention and deciding what you focus on.

We've already seen how ruminations and worry can end up making us anxious and harm our confidence. Meditation gives us the ability to decide what we want to think about – which can include not thinking about anything at all. Often, meditation amounts to simply calming your mind and clearing it. Once you get good, you can thus detach yourself from your thoughts or completely remove them at any given point.

The next time you are panicking about talking in public, you can simply choose to rise above it and let go of your anxiety – which is incredibly powerful.

Meditation also involves practiced breathing, which is one of the most effective ways to overcome stress. That's because our breathing is closely linked to our stress response and our sympathetic and parasympathetic nervous systems. When we're stressed, we breathe more rapidly to get more blood to our muscles and brain. When we slow down this breathing, it has the opposite effect and helps to move us back into the calmer state known as 'rest and digest'.

Over time, studies show that practicing meditation can help us to be calmer, happier and more logical. We can rise above things that don't matter and only focus on those things that do. Not only that, but it actually increases the dominance of slower, calmer brain waves. And it increases cortical thickness and the number of neural connections in the brain. In short, meditation is incredibly good for your brainpower and performance too.

So, contrary to popular beliefs, the benefits of meditation are evident in varying amounts immediately. Meditating every now and again is great and you'll see a change with every session that you do. However, a regular daily practice of meditation is the key to experiencing the full force of the exponentially increasing benefits.

How to Get Started with Meditation

The following four meditation techniques will help you to clear your mind and focus on visualizing confidence. They will help you to implant new belief systems into your subconscious and help you to think and act confidently.

1. Mindful Meditation

Mindfulness meditation is the practice of clearing your mind and focusing on nothing but the here and now without trying to change anything and without judgment. Engaging in this practice every day will allow you to control your stress and anxiety.

The more you work on it, the stronger your mindfulness power and endurance will become. When you are first starting a routine of mindfulness meditation, it is best to start with shorter amounts of time and increase your duration slowly. You also want to practice your meditation at the same time each day. The more you practice on a regular, consistent basis, the better the results.

Here are the steps to begin your daily practice of mindfulness meditation.

Step 1: Find a comfortable place to either sit up or lie straight. Sitting is often better because you are less likely to fall asleep.

Step 2: Set a timer. When you are first starting with your practice, it is better to keep your session around ten minutes. However, you can certainly increase this time if you feel you are able to sustain a more extended session.

Step 3: Begin taking calm breaths. Paying attention to how your breath feels going in your nose, down your lungs, and back out your nose. Pay attention to how your stomach or chest rises and falls with each breath. It is essential that you don't change your breathing or make any judgments. Breathe normally and merely focus on your breath and body.

Step 4: Next, you want to do a body scan. Start at the top of your head. Notice how it feels. Next, move down to your face. What does the back of your eyelids look like? How do your lips, nose, and chin feel Continue this process as you move down your entire body. Pay attention to feeling and temperature. Notice if there is any tightness or tension in your body, but don't try to change or fix any of the sensations. This process is about you merely noticing feelings and moving on.

Step 5: After you've completed the body scan, pay attention to the noises around you. First, notice the sounds of your body. Are you able to hear your breathing? Focus on just that sound. Next, focus on the sounds that are in the room. What noises are in the space? Then move onto the noises outside the space. What noises can you hear? Finally, focus your attention on the noises outside your living space. Can you hear anything?

Step 6: Finally, pay attention to how it feels to be in the moment. Let the thoughts that float into your mind float out again. Don't judge yourself for falling out of a mindfulness state and don't judge the thoughts that enter your mind. Don't attach any emotions to anything. Simply focus on each sensation that you feel.

Step 7: If you find one of the techniques works better for you, carry out the rest of your session using that technique, if not, just "be" until your timer rings.

2. Breathing Meditation

This technique helps to both focus and calm the mind, while physically relaxing the body. As with mindfulness meditation, you'll want to set a timer so that you can focus exclusively on your breathing without having to worry about the time.

Any time you feel overwhelmed, this technique can be extremely beneficial. It is effortless to practice because you can do it anywhere.

To prepare yourself for this meditation practice, you can either lie down or sit in a chair with your eyes open or closed. For a more profound relaxation, it is recommended that you sit or lie in a quiet space with your eyes closed.

Take deep inhales into your stomach, and fully exhale until you empty all the air from your lungs, making sure that each breath is rhythmic and consistent.

During this technique, inhale deeply until your belly rises and exhale fully as your stomach collapses and pulls in. The length of each breath isn't nearly as important as the consistency throughout your session.

3. Visualization

This kind of meditation practice will allow you to envision yourself acting confidently in all situations. You can use visualization before any significant event that causes you anxiety or use it daily to help you build your confidence over time. Follow the steps below to begin practicing visualization.

Step 1: Start your session with a few rounds of calm and controlled breathing. Only focus on your breath until both your body and mind become relaxed.

Step 2: Once you are in a relaxed state, say the following mantra: "I am confident" and feel confidence take over your entire being.

Step 3: In your mind, envision a clear, protective bubble forming around you. This is a shield where nothing negative can enter. Imagine that you are safe, secure, and radiating self-esteem in the bubble.

Step 4: Imagine your day ahead. Imagine that you are confidently approaching every situation, protected by this bubble of self-esteem. You walk with your head held high, interact with others confidently, speak assertively, and never doubt yourself.

Step 5: As you imagine each situation, continue to allow yourself to be filled with confidence. You visualize that you always know exactly what to say. Others see you as a successful and confident person. You are overflowing with happiness, positivity, and assurance.

Step 6: Continue this process until you have gone through every upcoming event. End the meditation session by affirming, "I will live this day radiating self-esteem and at peace with myself in all situations."

So the secret to properly visualizing is always to visualize what you want as if you had already achieved it. As opposed to hoping you'll achieve it or building confidence that one day it will occur, live and feel it as though it's happening to you today. On one level you understand that this is simply a psychological trick, but the subconscious mind can't differentiate between what's real and what is imagined. Your subconscious will act upon the pictures you create inside, whether they represent your present reality or not.

4. Anchoring

Anchoring is a Neuro-Linguistic Programming technique that is used to induce a frame of mind or emotion. It is a conditioning that forms when a person evokes a feeling and pairs it with a gesture or touch of some kind.

To practice this technique, you need to get into a meditative state.

Use mindfulness, breathing, or any combination to start. Then, you want to think of an emotion that you want to condition; it can be success, confidence, relaxation, or happiness. Now, picture a time in your life when you experienced the desired emotion.

If you aspire to feel confident, think of a time in your past when you experienced confidence. Perhaps, it was when you received the top grade in a class, or when your high school football team won the state championship.

Picture in your mind that moment and experience the emotions as if they are currently happening. While feeling the emotion, hold your index finger and thumb together. Relax for a few seconds, then reimagine the experience with a heightened state of feeling and bring your thumb and index finger together again.

Repeat this process three to five times. By repeating this exercise daily, when you put your thumb and index finger together, eventually you'll experience the same emotion, no matter the circumstance.

You can use this technique to recondition your thinking. For example, if you anchor a feeling of confidence, anytime you experience feelings of overwhelm or doubt, you can use this anchor to stimulate a positive, confident state.

Anchoring can also be used with other visualization techniques as well. For instance, once you have set your anchor, you can visualize being confident in your current or future pursuits. Engage the anchor by merely placing your index finger and thumb together and experience the emotional response of confidence, making your visualization more real.

Chapter 8

How to Use Affirmations Effectively for Solid Confidence

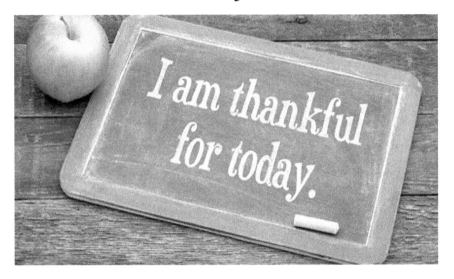

Affirmations are self-talk statements & better presented to the subconscious. These fresh images are viewed as "credible" by the subconscious & are placed in the area of subconscious having to do with the power to enhance the ability to pull up particular powerful memories with less work.

Through this special imagery, a person can develop the inner tools for the correct mindset for gaining confidence, letting the memories and images be transported to the here and now where they're used for enhancing mindset which is crucial for concrete confidence.

Affirmations might help you to change adverse behaviors or achieve the correct mindset, and they can likewise help undo the harm caused by negative scripts, those things which we repeatedly tell ourselves that add to a negative self-perception and affect our success.

Now that you understand the importance of the affirmations, let's see how to use them to get the best result with the least effort.

How to use affirmations

A powerful way to jump in using affirmations for concrete confidence is to write them down on an index card, and read it throughout the day. The more you practice them, the deeper the new beliefs will click. The best times to review your affirmations are first thing in the morning time, during the day, and prior to you retiring for the night.

But let's see in more detail how to maximize their effectiveness by applying these practical tips:

- Use affirmations while meditating. After relaxing into a deep, quiet, meditative frame of mind, imagine that you're you have already become confident and know how to manage any situation. Imagine yourself in the physical setting or environment that you would like, the house that you enjoy and find comforting, drawing in loads of people into your life and receiving appreciation and appropriate financial recompense for your efforts. Add any other details that are essential for you, like the promotion you want, the people you want to meet monthly, and so forth. Try to get a feeling in yourself that this is possible; experience it like it was already happening. In brief, imagine it exactly the way you'd like it to be as if it were already so!

- Try standing in front of a mirror and use affirmations while looking into your own eyes. If you can, repeat them out loud with passion. This is a powerful way to change your limiting beliefs very quickly.

- If you find it hard to believe an affirmation will happen, add "I choose to" to the affirmation. "I choose to be more confident," for instance, or, "I choose to get a promotion."

- Make a recording in your own voice and play it as you doze off. Some individuals swear by this technique.

- Attach positive emotions to your affirmations. Consider how achieving your goal will make you feel, or consider how good it feels to know that you're succeeding at becoming more confident. Emotion is a fuel that makes affirmations more potent.

- If you don't want people to know about your confidence affirmations, simply place your reminders in discreet locations. Remember, however, that it's essential that you see them frequently, or they'll do you no good.

- If you find yourself merely parroting the words of your affirmations, instead of focusing on their meaning, change affirmations. You're able to still affirm the same goals or characteristics, naturally, but rephrasing your affirmations can regenerate their effectiveness.

Well, now that you know the best ways and moments to use affirmations, the next step will be to create your own statements. Here's how to do it.

Create your own affirmations

- Consider your positive attributes. Take stock of yourself by making a list of your best qualities, abilities, or additional properties. Are you adept at meeting new people? Write it down. Are you a good speaker? Make mention of it. Write each quality down in a brief sentence, starting with "I" and using the present tense: "I'm adept at meeting new people," for example, or "I'm a good speaker ". These statements are affirmations of who you are. We seldom revolve around those things that we sincerely like about ourselves, rather choosing to dwell on things we don't like. A list will help you break up that cycle, and using these affirmations to help you appreciate who you are will give you the confidence you need to accept your affirmations.

- Consider what negative scripts you'd like to neutralize or what positive confidence goals you'd like to achieve. Affirmations can be highly useful to counteract negative perceptions you have acquired about your abilities to be confident or make a success out of a new venture. Affirmations may also help you accomplish specific goals, like meeting new people or achieving a successful business. Make a list of your goals or the adverse self-percepts you'd like to alter.

- Prioritize your list of matters to work on. You may find that you have a lot of goals or that you require many different affirmations. It's best, though, to revolve around just a couple of affirmations at once, so pick those that are most crucial or most urgent and work with those first of all. When you see improvement in those areas or achieve those goals you can phrase new affirmations for other points on your list.

- Use positive affirmations alone as counter-scripts, or add other affirmations to mold your behavior with and about your confidence in the future. The affirmations you'll use to mold future changes should follow the same form. They should begin with "I," and be curt, clear, and positive. There are 2 forms of future-oriented affirmations you can utilize to work toward goals.

- "I can" statements: author a statement affirming the fact that you can accomplish your goal(s). For example, if you'd like to date a new person, a statement like "I can date a new person," is a good start. Several experts recommend that you avoid any form of negative connotation.
- "I will" statements: author a statement affirming that today you'll really utilize your ability to accomplish your goal. So, following the above example, you may say, "I will date a new person. Again, the affirmation should use positive language and should plainly express what you'll do today to accomplish the longer-term goal of being more confident.

- Match-up a few of your positive attributes with your goals. Which of the positive characters will help you accomplish the goals you've set? If you're addressing ways to speak to new people, for instance, you may need bravery or courage. Select affirmations to support what you'll need.
- Make your repetitions visible so you'll be able to utilize them. Repetition is the key to making affirmations effective. You want to consider your affirmations several times a day, daily.

- Proceed using your affirmations. The more you affirm something, the more steadfastly your mind will accept it. If you're trying to accomplish a short-term goal, use your affirmations till you've accomplished it. If you merely want to use affirmations as a counter-script, practice each one as long as you like.

Examples of Affirmations

To make your work easier, here is an example list of positive affirmations that work and that you can use for starting:

1. *I believe in my abilities and skills;*
2. *My mistakes are seen as growing and learning opportunities;*
3. *I am constantly seeking growth to better myself;*
4. *I have power over my emotions, they do not control me;*
5. *I am a fearless leader;*
6. *I attract loving relationships because I am being myself and people love that about me*
7. *I am a powerhouse of productivity*
8. *I believe in myself so deeply*
9. *I achieve everything that my soul is aligned with*
10. *I combat negative thoughts with empowering thoughts*
11. *Confidence comes natural to me*
12. *I learn and grow daily*
13. *I have the power to change myself*

14. *I have rock solid belief in myself and my ability to succeed*

15. *My mind is wide open to all the possibilities around me*

16. *I face my fears, allowing me to become more powerful and creating even more self-belief;*

17. *My power is unlimited;*

18. *I accept that I cannot change the past. I focus on my future and move forward in my life. My past does not define who I am today.*

19. *I trust my own wisdom and intuition. I am the only person who knows what is best for me.*

20. *My voice matters and I am confident to speak up when I want to. People listen to me because my words are valuable.*

Each one of these affirmations will help you regain your self-confidence in any situation or in any field.

Believing in yourself is a daily journey. And in this path, the single words, as well as the phrases, have their importance not to be underestimated.

Chapter 9

How to Set and Achieve All Your Goals

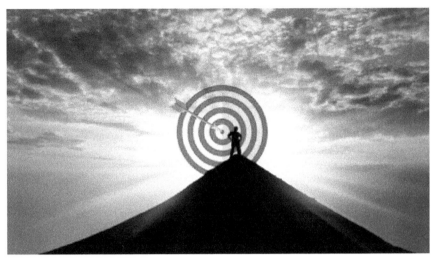

Nobody is born knowing exactly how to set goals or how to achieve the things they desire in life. Like with other things, goal setting is an art that needs to be learned and perfected. Reaching goals is a crucial part of strengthening self-confidence: it helps shape and updates exactly how you define yourself while at the same time helping you add to your sense of accomplishment.

In addition, setting your goals will give you a long-term vision and short-term motivation.

More specifically, the setting of goals is a very important method for:

- Deciding what you want to achieve in your life.
- Separating what's important from what's irrelevant
- Motivating yourself.

- Building your self-confidence, based on the successful achievement of goals.

A useful way to make goals more powerful and improve personal productivity is to use the **SMART method**.

SMART means:

S – Specific

M – Measurable

A – Attainable

R – Relevant

T – Time-bound (or Trackable).

The S.M.A.R.T. method was developed by Peter Drucker in 1954. It is a system for the identification, definition, and pursuit of specific and quantifiable objectives.

Let's see how it works and we analyze each point in detail.

How to Use SMART approach for goals achievement

1. Specific

Your goal should be clear and specific, otherwise, you won't be able to focus your efforts or feel truly motivated to achieve it. When drafting your goal, try to answer the following questions:

- What do I want to accomplish?
- Why is this goal important?
- Who is involved?
- Where is it located?
- Which resources or limits are involved?

The more specific you can be in the description of what you want to achieve, the higher the chances you will be able to reach it.

2. Measurable

It's important to have measurable goals so that you can track your progress and stay motivated. Assessing progress helps you to stay focused, meet your deadlines, and feel the excitement of getting closer to achieving your goal.

A measurable goal should address questions such as:

- How much?
- How many?
- How will I know when it is accomplished?

3. Achievable

Your goal also needs to be realistic and attainable to be successful. In other words, it should stretch your abilities but still remain possible. When you set an achievable goal, you may be able to identify previously overlooked opportunities or resources that can bring you closer to it.

An achievable goal will usually answer questions such as:

- How can I accomplish this goal?
- How realistic is the goal, based on other constraints, such as financial factors?

This does not mean that you have to choose goals that are too small, easy to achieve or insignificant: the best solution is in the middle.

You need to set goals big enough to get you excited and motivated to improve, but small enough to be possible and achievable.

4. Relevant

This step is about ensuring that your goal matters to you and that it also aligns with other relevant goals. We all need support and assistance in achieving our goals, but it's important to retain control over them. So, make sure that your plans drive everyone forward, but that you're still responsible for achieving your own goal.

A relevant goal can answer "yes" to these questions:

- Does this seem worthwhile?
- Is this the right time?
- Does this match our other efforts/needs?
- Am I the right person to reach this goal?
- Is it applicable in the current socio-economic environment?

5. Time-bound

Every goal needs a target date so that you have a deadline to focus on and something to work toward. This part of the SMART goal criteria helps to prevent everyday tasks from taking priority over your longer-term goals.

A time-bound goal will usually answer these questions:

- When?
- What can I do six months from now?
- What can I do six weeks from now?

- What can I do today?

Along the way, there will be obstacles to overcome and unforeseen events that could waste your time, keep this in mind when associating a date with a goal.

Finally, remember the most important thing: celebrate when you have reached a goal in the timeframe you set.

Examples of smart targets

Now that you know what a smart goal is, we'll see together some examples of successful planning using SMART goals.

NON-SMART GOALS	SMART GOALS
Be in good physical shape	*Lose 10 kg by 1 July*
Having a salary increase	*Have an increase of 200 euros by 1 October*
Learn English well	*Passing the TOEFL exam on September 16*
Become a writer	*Publish a book before the end of the year*

As you can see, the goals on the left are very vague, generic, without expiration and absolutely no measurable. The goals on the right, instead, are much more precise, motivating and achievable. In short... they push you into action! And this is precisely the main function of a goal.

Other basic tips

In addition to the SMART approach, if you want to achieve your goals you will also need to follow these 3 significant suggestions:

1. Write Them Down

Writing your goals down ensures that you think through every little detail and how each task will be actualized to eventually accomplish the goal. It also ensures that you can remember your goals because research has shown a strong correlation between writing and memory retention.

2. Track Your Goals Regularly

It is important that you track your goals regularly on a weekly or monthly basis. Look back on where you come from and observe those small wins you needed on the journey. Don't take these tiny successes for granted and in no way let them go undetected.

Every time you accomplish any of these goals, your brain will be conditioned to focus on what matters most and start achieving more!

3. Visualize

The other important tip is for you to picture yourself having attained the goals. Studies have demonstrated that the motor parts of the brain will be activated when you perform the tasks physically. One study had two groups; one that practiced the piano physically and another that played piano mentally.

The most interesting thing was that those that practiced through visualization were just as effective as those that practiced physically. Meaning you don't have to physically practice something to get good at something. This study explains the power of visualization and you too should use visualization to get better at any skill or achieve any goal.

Stop Procrastinating on Your Goals

Many times, we have resistance against the action and change when we need those two most. You require a little bit of discipline, but the benefits of quitting to put off things are massive.

Putting off things makes them tougher and scarier. There's nothing worse and more trying than the lingering of unfinished jobs. It is like an extra weight in your shoulder which does not allow you to enjoy what you're doing. It merely causes stress.

The majority of the time you'll come to realize the things you procrastinated can really be accomplished very quickly with the advantage that subsequently you are feeling much lighter and will forget about it.

Procrastinating is avoiding something which should be done. It's putting off things hoping they get better without really doing anything about them. The issue is that most of the time things do not get better on their own; they get worse.

Many times, the reason behind procrastination is fear.
Another source is feeling overwhelmed.

You're procrastinating when you're...

- ...doing nothing rather than what it is you're supposed to do.
- ...doing something less important than what you should do.
- ...doing something more significant than what we're meant to do.

The key to getting started is simply that. Get started.
Normally, by beginning, you build enough momentum to keep continuing. Simply focus on taking the first step. And then another. And another. These tiny steps will add up to results fairly quickly.

The only difference between people who reach their targets and those who do not, between successful and unsuccessful people is 1 thing: Taking action. A year from now you'll thank you for getting started now.

The only difference between that which you want to be and that you are now is what you do from now onwards. Your activities will take you there. It will not be easy. There'll be a pain, you'll require willpower, dedication, patience and you should make some challenging decisions. You might even need to let some folks go. Many times it is going to be much easier to give up.

You will be tempted to give up several times, but remember one thing: When you reach your goal it'll be worth all the sacrifice. "Is it worthwhile to be bombarded by and lose my sleep over a job that I could have completed in a couple of hours?" The best time to begin any endeavor is always NOW! By putting together all these suggestions you will be able to plan and fulfill your goals, thus increasing your confidence as well.

Chapter 10

How to Face and Overcome a Failure

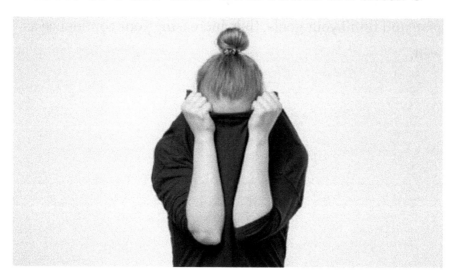

Things often don't go well. You make a mistake, have a setback or you simply fail. It's no fun. But you can't avoid it either unless you avoid doing anything at all. So it is necessary to learn how to handle these situations by avoiding being drawn into negativity.

"It doesn't matter IF you fall, or WHY, but HOW YOU REACT to the falls"

Failure is an essential condition for any great success. If you want to succeed quickly, start collecting failures right away. Have you ever watched a child learn to walk or cycle? Stumble and fall countless times before you reach your coveted goal.

Children show us that mistakes are learning opportunities. And that failure is necessary if we are to achieve success. Here are 9 simple reminders not to be forgotten after an error or failure.

1. Accept Failure

Even though failure is truly unpleasant, you have to understand that it is an opportunity to learn. When you are trying to create something, you need to accept the fact that things will never be perfect, and that is why failures are bound to happen from time to time.

From every failure, ask yourself what can you learn from it, and what will you do differently next time. This will ensure that you can implement proper strategies in your next project to ensure that these things do not happen again. One of the greatest lessons you can learn is how to fail gracefully. This way, you get to learn the necessary lessons to boost your ability to innovate.

2. There is no success without failure.

A person who does not make mistakes will be able to achieve few goals in his life. It is not a paradox: only those who have the courage to take risks and make mistakes can go far. Those who are afraid of making mistakes will be careful and will probably never fail, but will not go far.

It is preferable to have a life full of small failures from which to draw important lessons, rather than a life full of regrets for not even trying.

3. Accept your emotions.

You're not a slave to your emotions - even though it sometimes feels like it. You're the only one responsible for your own emotions. It is not others that cause your emotions; it is your response to what others do or say.

Your emotions come from your ideas, and you have learned by now that you could train to control your own thoughts. An emotion is a power in movement, a physical response to a thought.

You do not have to be scared of your own emotions. They're part of you, but they're not you. Emotions are merely that, and every emotion has its own function.

There is nothing terrible about being sad, frustrated, angry or envious every now and then, but as soon as you notice this sort of emotion creeping up inside you, analyze where it comes from.

Become an observer and see where your emotions lead you. Watch them like the clouds in a blue sky. Accept them as if you accept rainy days. When you check from the window, and it rains you accept that the rain as part of the meteorological climate, right? -- You know it does not mean that it will rains all of the time. Just because they appear at one moment in time does not mean that they'll be there forever.

Learn how to handle your emotions that means perceive, use, understand, and manage them. It is done as follows:

1. Perceive and express emotions and allow yourself to feel them.
2. Facilitation of feelings. Ask yourself how you can feel a different emotion.
3. Understand the emotion is coming up. There is always a motive and an inherent belief.
4. Emotional modification. You understand the reason emotion was felt.

Managing your emotions has enormous advantages: You recover faster and better from problems and drawbacks. You're able to protect against those anxieties from building up to ruin your relationships. You regulate your impulses and contradictory emotions. You remain balanced and calm even in crucial moments.

Just because today is painful does not mean that tomorrow will not be great. You just have to persevere, don't give up. The best things usually happen when you least expect it. And in the meantime, try to smile, it will be worth the effort.

4. Positive thinking creates positive results.

If you don't like something, change it. If you can't change it, change your way of thinking, look at reality from a different perspective. There is always an angle from which things look rosier, more positive. Not to cry on yourself is a choice completely in your hands.

Winston Churchill said, "Success is passing from one failure to another without losing enthusiasm." The mind must believe that it can do something before it can actually do it. Negative thinking creates negative results, it is true, but the opposite is also true: positive thinking creates positive results.

5. Success is always closer than it seems.

Make your mistakes and failures your motivation, not your excuse. Mistakes teach you important lessons. Whenever you commit one, you are one step closer to your goal.

The only mistake that can really hurt you is the choice to do nothing because you are too afraid to make mistakes. Failure is not a fall down, but the exciting run-up before an exciting ascent.

6. You are not your mistakes.

Together with the life you have not been given the instruction booklet. Accept the fact that you will make mistakes, just like everyone else.

You are not your mistakes, do not identify with them: at any time you have the opportunity to throw your mistakes behind you, shape your reality and decide your tomorrow.

No matter how complex and painful the past was, the future is pristine, pure, a window wide open to your successes: what to do with it depends only on you.

7. The most important life lessons are learned in unexpected moments.

We don't look for many of the greatest lessons we learn in life. In reality, we learn the most important lessons in the worst moments and from the biggest mistakes.

So yes, it's true, sometimes you'll be wrong, but that's okay. The faster you accept this fact, the faster you will reach your goals.

8. Mistakes are rarely as serious as they seem.

Failures, errors, and setbacks are rarely as relevant as they may seem at first sight. And even when they are, they give us the opportunity to become stronger.

You should never let a single dark cloud let us see the whole sky covered. The sun always shines somewhere in your life. Sometimes it is enough to forget how you feel, remember what you deserve, and keep on going with a smile.

9. You have the ability to create your own happiness.

You can decide to remain anchored in the mistakes of the past, or you can decide to create your own happiness for the present and the future. A smile is a choice, not a miracle. Don't make the mistake of waiting for someone or something to come to you to make you happy.

You are primarily responsible for your own happiness. Inner peace begins when you choose not to allow external events and situations to control your emotions.

10. Life goes on.

Mistakes are painful when they occur, but years later, this collection of errors, called experience, will be what will have led you to success. Everything that goes wrong is experience anyway. Your mentality is at the center of your success. Always welcome with a smile the good and bad things that happen to you during your life.

Love what you have and be grateful for what you have had. Forgive yourself and others, but don't forget. Learn from your mistakes, but don't feel sorry for yourself. Life is change, things sometimes go wrong, but life goes on. And you accompany it with a smile.

Chapter 11

Building Your Social Confidence (Overcoming Social Anxiety and Be bulletproof)

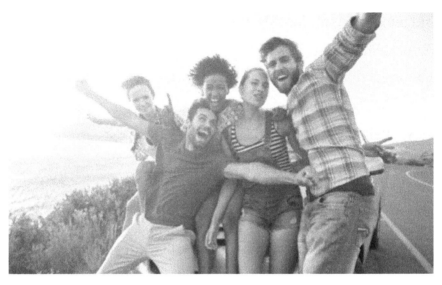

We all want people to like us, but for that to happen we have to improve our social confidence.

Knowing how to make new friends and how to feel confident around strangers is very important to your self-esteem and emotional well-being. But there are many things that might be holding you back. And among the most common issues in this regard, is social anxiety.

What is social anxiety?

Social anxiety is the fear of being judged and evaluated negatively by others, resulting in feelings of inadequacy, inferiority, self-consciousness, embarrassment, humiliation, and depression.

Social anxiety prevents individuals from expressing their ideas and temperament, for this, they usually are misunderstood. People with social anxiety disorder experience significant emotional distress in the following situations:

- Being introduced to other people;
- Being teased or criticized;
- Being the center of attention;
- Being watched while doing something;
- Meeting important people;
- Most social encounters, especially with strangers;
- Going around the room (or table) in a circle and having to say something;
- Interpersonal relationships, whether friendships or romantic;

This list is certainly not a complete list of symptoms, other feelings have been associated with social anxiety as well.

Where Does Social Anxiety Come from?

Experts today part with some of the ideas of earlier decades in believing most cases of Social Anxiety disorder don't spring from one event lasting effects, but instead, Social Anxiety is the result of a number of different probable causes. These can include both environmental and genetic factors.

Here are some of the most prominent of the factors leading to Social Anxiety disorder.

1. Genetic Roots

Social Anxiety disorder has been shown to run in family lines. Recent research has shown that this is not just learned behavior, but almost certainly also has genetic origins.

2. Over Developed Amygdala

The amygdala is the part of the brain responsible for the fear response. When it is overdeveloped leads to an increased tendency towards Social Anxiety disorder.

3. Unbalanced Serotonin Levels

Serotonin is a key brain chemical that regulates emotional states. When unbalanced Social Anxiety disorder can become the end result. This can come from natural causes or have become unbalanced from past drug or alcohol abuse.

4. Family Conflict

A history of family conflict, especially at an early age, is one of the most common social factors known to cause Social Anxiety disorder.

5. Bullying

Bullying is one of the environmental factors that has been receiving a great deal of attention lately for it being known to aggravate young people's Social Anxiety sometimes with very tragic results.

6. **History of Sexual Abuse or Extreme Maltreatment**

Sexual abuse and other severe maltreatment very often lead to the more severe end of Social Anxiety disorder. In many cases, these types of experiences require multiple levels of therapy to ultimately resolve not only the heightened social anxiety but also the other effects of this trauma.

Sometimes determining its root can be difficult. Thankfully the methods used to cure it have been shown to be effective regard

How to Overcome Social Anxiety using Cognitive Restructuring

Cognitive restructuring, in essence, means that you are 'reprogramming' the way that you interpret events and the way that you think about future events.

Cognitive restructuring generally incorporates two main components. These are 'thought challenging' and 'hypothesis testing'.

Thought challenging means that you are going to be looking at the things you are visualizing and the things you are telling yourself and then you are going to restructure your mindset by challenging those beliefs – by testing them for validity.

So, for example, you might be telling yourself that if you speak up in public, people will ignore you and you will look foolish. But now ask yourself this:

- Are these people not your friends?
- And therefore, is it really likely they'd ignore you?
- Moreover, would it really matter?
- If they're not your friends, are you even ever going to see them again?
- Isn't it better to at least try?

These days, the likelihood of being ostracized socially and left to fend for ourselves in the wild is highly unlikely. Meaning that it is pretty safe to speak up in any setting, no matter who you are!

And remember, we have the tendency to inflate the risk and minimize reward. So be honest with yourself and rational and you can normally reduce the fear and the anxiety.

Hypothesis testing meanwhile means that you are going to literally test the theory and prove to yourself that there is nothing to be afraid of. Prove to yourself that you don't need to be worried about getting laughed at.

So this might mean that you intentionally say something stupid, just to see how people react. Or how about you purposefully go to say something in public and then stutter. What you'll find is that most people are patient and understanding and will react by simply waiting for you to finish. They'll even give you a big, support round of applause. In short, hypothesis testing means facing your fears head-on and seeing that they aren't so bad. And what's more, is that by repeatedly facing your fears. By repeatedly putting yourself in frightening scenarios, you can actually become desensitized to the fear. If you keep speaking up in public, then you'll find that you eventually normalize it and it no longer becomes a big deal.

You can practice this in several ways:

- Strike up conversations with strangers wherever possible
- Talk to shop tenders – be purposefully awkward or strange in places where you don't need to come back!
- Ask people for their numbers
- Make complaints if you aren't happy with customer service
- Attend stand-up comedy classes, acting classes or singing lessons. Anything where you have to perform in front of people

Do all this, and over time you'll become more and more calm. You won't have the fight or flight response when you talk or perform in public and as such, you'll come across as much more confident.

People will assume that means you have absolute faith in what you're doing, or that you're secretly rich or incredibly ripped. But in reality, you have just learned not to fret the small stuff.

How to Create a Good First Impression

This is especially important because those first impressions mean a great deal. The way you impact someone when you first meet them makes a huge impact on your overall confidence, esteem, and importance in their eyes.

So, practice making that great first impression. That means walking with powerful strides and beaming into the room and it means shaking their hand firmly and with purpose. If you want to seem confident and make the best first impression then there are few things worse than a limp, wet fish handshake!

1. Eye Contact

Another key component of creating a good impression when you first meet someone and conveying confidence is maintaining proper eye contact. Holding eye contact suggests that you feel equal to the person you're speaking to and it gives you more intensity, makes you seem more honest and in other words sends all of those good social signals that we want to send!

So, try to maintain good eye contact but without being creepy. Hold the gaze for a few seconds, then look away while gesticulating and then hold the gaze again. And when speaking in front of a larger group, make sure that you look around the group and remember to hold eye contact with each person for a few seconds.

2. Speak More Slowly

One of the things that will help you to seem more confident while communicating is to speak more slowly. We are naturally inclined to speed up as we become nervous and this can lead to us stumbling over our words and seeming less confident and less sure of what we're saying. Of course, this is not good!

On the other hand, if you speak more slowly, then you come across as someone who knows what they're talking about, who is confident in who they are and who has thought about what they're saying. Because you're giving yourself time, you'll also be less likely to stutter or to pause and need to use um, filler words.

3. Tell Stories

Telling stories also conveys confidence. And this works in tandem with speaking more slowly.

One of the reasons we speak quickly when we are talking in public is to get it over with more quickly. We speak quickly because

a) we aren't naturally fond of talking in public and we want it to stop and...

b) we aren't confident that what we're saying is compelling enough or interesting enough and we're worried that people will stop listening if we don't finish what we're saying quickly!

But if you tell a story then this suggests that you are more natural when it comes to holding court and entertaining a crowd. It suggests you're enjoying it and that you have confidence in your own ability to entertain.

And this effect is felt even more strongly if you slow it down. Not only in terms of how you speak but also in your delivery. That means that you set the scene, you ask rhetorical questions, you use repetition and you create suspense.

This is something that most charismatic people can pull off tremendously and it has a huge impact when done well. Don't rush to the point, enjoy the moment, linger and have faith in how interesting you are!

Nobody is better than you!

. . .and you're also not better than others. You're different. You're fantastic, but it doesn't mean that you are better than others. It doesn't imply that others cannot be great, also, in their own special way. Your greatness doesn't take away the greatness of others.

We were brought up with the mindset that others that have a name, a particular social position, or even more cash are superior to us and we must admire them.

Everything is going so quickly nowadays. Titles and status do not mean so much anymore. For example, there are lots of people with a college or even doctorate title that's jobless; on the other hand, some of the best companies in the world have been built by people who did not finish school or even high school.

On the one hand, individuals lose societal positions while others proceed upward. They're different, but it doesn't mean they're better than you. Bear in mind that.

Reconnect with Friends to Build Your Self-Confidence

You may be thinking, what do friends have to do with self-confidence? Each one of us has moments of self-doubt and insecurities. It is very common to be anxious about our looks. Often times, you may find yourself questioning whether you said the right thing or did the right thing in any given situation. Sometimes, it is something as minor as matching your dress with the right pair of shoes, or your shirt with the right tie.

Just like any other person, when I am not sure of these things, I turn to my friends for a second opinion. One thing that you may have noticed is that certain people play a very important role in building our confidence. It is through friends that we can shake that skepticism or uncertainty we have about ourselves. It is through them that we can make better decisions in life.

These are some of the ways reconnecting with friends helps build up our confidence:

They Cheer for Your Success

If there is someone that you call when you have good news to share, it is your friend. Friends are among the first few groups of people we can go to when we have problems, frustrations or setbacks. The main reason is that they take pride in what we accomplish. They are the people that cheer us on and believe in us that we can do it! Knowing that someone's got your back will help you face anything with so much confidence.

They Model New Ways of Being

No man is perfect, so the saying goes. However, with friends, they also have strengths and skills that help them perform better in what they do. I have a friend that moves the crowd with his speech. At some point, I wondered whether I might do the same.

With a model to look up to, it became a lot easier to move towards your goal. By simply modeling his way of giving a speech, I became better eventually. The same thing applies to you; having a friend helps us see ways we can use their strengths to improve our areas of weakness.

They Support Our Efforts to Grow

Did you know that sometimes the only thing that stands between you and your success is your mindset? Well, now, you do. The reason why you have cold feet about going after that business idea is that your thoughts are telling you that you cannot do it.

However, when you surround yourself with positive friends, they can see strengths in you that you never knew existed.

That will give you enough motivation to give it a try, and you realize that you just needed a little push to soar like an eagle.

They Wipe Our Tears Away

In this journey called life, there will always be bumps along the road. It can be failing an exam, losing a tournament, being dumped or even worse losing a loved one. However, when you have friends, you have someone to lean on to when you're down.

They will be there to give you insights from a different perspective. They will bring so much sunshine to your darkest moments.

They Teach Us the Value of Teamwork

Confidence is not just about working alone. It is about knowing how to walk the road alone and when to walk it with a team. Sometimes, when you are alone, you may feel timid and insecure about going to places or try new things or do things differently.

However, if you are doing those things with a friend, there is a sudden splash of energy, and you realize that you can become creative. This allows you to soar higher than you had dreamed possible.

The truth is, the very best part of reconnecting with friends is the fact that feelings are reciprocal. They are the people that share our dreams, and we can do the same for them. So, surround yourself with true friends and see how that impacts your attitude and confidence to stretch beyond limits.

Chapter 12

Boost Your Self-Confidence with Your Body Language

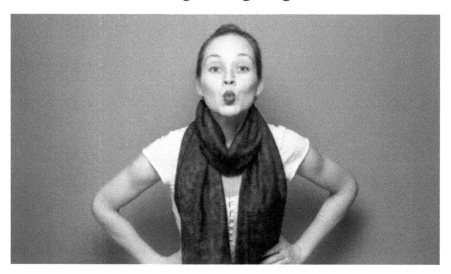

Your body language is one of the single most important tools for conveying the way you feel. Communication is often estimated as being 70% non-verbal or even higher. In other words, what you're saying with your mouth is far less important than what you say with your body. You can talk the talk, but if you're hunched up, then you will convey a sense of anxiety and low confidence.

The good news is that even if you don't feel confident, practicing confident body language can increase your self-esteem and make you feel better about yourself.

Your brain and body language communicate with one another constantly. And this communication is a 2-way street. One on end, your body language is reflecting the thoughts and feelings going on in your mind. But at the same time, the thoughts and feelings you have are influenced by the messages your brain gets from your body language. This means that by adopting positive body language you can actually become a more confident man.

So how do you fix your body language?

To learn how to take advantage of this psychological phenomenon, check out the tips below on how to build confidence through body language.

1. Smile to be happy

Smiling is perhaps the most confident thing you can do. Want to look more confident when you walk? Then smile as you go! Want to look more confident when approaching members of the opposite sex in a bar? Just smile at them from across the room and you'll not only appear friendly, but also as though you're happy to make yourself vulnerable – which again makes you seem relaxed and confident.

Smiling actually makes us feel more confident too due to a psychological phenomenon known as 'facial feedback'. This means that we will often feel the way we look. Smile and you feel happier. Grimace and you feel angrier. Smiling in particular releases serotonin which induces feel-good feels. Even if the smile is forced, it still works!

2. Posture

The body language communication you have with your brain isn't limited to the messages sent from your face. Your brain is actually picking up messages from all over your body to determine how you should be feeling. So if you want to feel more positive and confident, you've got to send messages of confidence from the rest of your body as well.

To send those messages make sure to keep your head up, shoulders rolled down and back, and your spine straight – as if there's a string pulling from the base of your spine up through the crown of your head. At the same time let your muscles relax and focus on taking slow breathes deep into the belly. Adopting this posture while breathing deeply and relaxing your muscles will send signals of confidence to your brain. You'll start to feel more relaxed and self-assured as a result.

3. Walk with confidence

The body language communication we've been discussing is always in play – even when you're walking. Our walk says a lot about us and if we walk briskly, powerfully and proudly, then we can make ourselves seem confident, large and in charge before we even start speaking!

Conversely, if we walk in a slumped, hunched and shuffling manner, then we will just seem shy, retiring and scared.

To walk taller, the trick that is often described is to imagine that a beam of light is bursting out from your chest. That means you're walking with your chest slightly poised upwards and it means that you should be smiling and walking briskly. The problem is remembering to do this! Most of us have been walking pretty regularly now since we were... well one year old! Thus it's hard to just drop those years of ingrained training and start walking in a wholly different way.

A way around this is to look for triggers to remind you. One of the best of these is walking through a doorway. The next time you cross a threshold, use this as a way to remember that trick and start beaming again.

4. Power poses

Just as smiling can work in reverse to change your emotions, so too does your body language influence the way you feel. When we are confident, we have a tendency to take up more space. What you might not realize is that when you take up more space, it makes you feel more confident.

Why? Because it triggers a rush of the hormone testosterone, testosterone being the primary male hormone and also a neurotransmitter that increases aggression and assertiveness. Psychologists have thus managed to find what is known as power positions. These are positions you can pull with your body that will instantly make you feel more confident and on top of the world.

The most well-known of these is the victory position. Simply hold your hands over your head in a v shape as you might when crossing the finish line victorious in a race. This is a universal position in fact and is something that people do across cultures – even apes are thought to use this signal to demonstrate victory and success!

And apparently, it triggers an immediate increase in testosterone. So the next time you're about to do an interview or go on a date, try going to the toilet first and practicing a few power positions!

5. Open up your body language

Another way for body language communication to send messages of confidence to your brain is from keeping your body language open. Keep your arms by your side and don't use them to cover yourself up (avoid crossing your arms or holding a drink across your chest). Crossing your arms is a defensive posture and sends signals to your brain that there's a need to protect yourself. Keeping your arms by your side however, tells your brain you have nothing to fear.

In addition to keeping your arms uncrossed, don't cross your legs when standing. Instead stand with your legs apart (hip to shoulder width) and maintain a strong, solid base. Don't be afraid to take up a bit of room and really own the space around you. Adopting this kind of body language communicates feelings of strength and power directly to your brain.

Another body language trick is to try leaning on things. If you lean against a wall, this communicates ownership. Likewise, if you touch someone on the shoulder, this conveys a kind of ownership which also comes across as confidence.

6. Gesticulate

Speaking of the most charismatic people, science also has something to say about this topic.

In studies, it has been shown that people who are rated as the most charismatic, also tend to gesticulate the most. Gesticulation means talking with your hands, it means being animated and pointing, gesturing and pacing around as you speak. And the reason that this is associated with confidence and charisma, is because it makes us seem more engaged with what we ourselves are saying. Now our body language and our words are congruent and our passion can, therefore, be felt around the room.

The more you gesture as you speak, the more passionate and emphatic you seem to be about what you're saying. And this is highly engaging and impressive – it makes everyone else perceive it as more engaging and interesting too!

Avoid negative body language

Your brain isn't just picking up on positive body language communication signals. It's picking up on the negative ones, too. So if you indulge in negative, insecure body language, you're communicating to your brain that you should be feeling negative and insecure. Negative feelings will arise and be reinforced anytime you maintain negative body language.

So don't just embrace the confident, positive body language mentioned above, but make a point to avoid the opposite body language. If you catch yourself frowning, slumping your shoulders, shuffling your feet, or making yourself "small", take note and immediately adopt the opposite behavior. This will help you spark more positive feelings and gradually move out of that negative state of mind.

Don't Fidget

Fidgeting is a clear sign of nervousness. A man who can't keep still is a man who is worried, tense and certainly not confident. Your hands can be your worst enemies -- fight to keep them still and steady. You can definitely talk with your hands but keep your gesticulations calm and under control. Also, when seated, avoid that rapid leg-vibration thing that some guys do (you don't want to look like a dog getting his belly rubbed). When we're nervous or stressed, we all pacify with some form of self-touching, nonverbal behavior: We rub our hands together, bounce our feet, drum our fingers on the desk, play with our jewelry, twirl our hair, fidget — and when we do any of these things, we immediately rob our statements of credibility.

Chapter 13

How to Get a Physique That Will Make You Confident

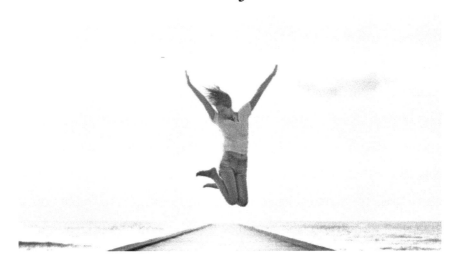

The best ways to enhance your confidence are those that we've discussed already. These address the deep-seated causes for low esteem and they help you to train yourself out of panic and anxiety responses.

That means improving yourself, finding role models, reminding yourself of positive interactions and successes, surrounding yourself with the right people, facing your fears and practicing being social. Finally, find your passion and invest in that, without worrying about what others think.

All this does a great deal to enhance your esteem But, in the meantime, that isn't to say that there aren't smaller and easier changes you can make to boost your esteem. And sometimes, this means focusing on the external aspect. It means looking at surface-level aspects of yourself that you might not be happy in.

Many of us have low self-esteem primarily because we don't like the way we look or because we think we are out of shape. If you are overweight, overly thin or conventionally unattractive, then this can make it hard to overlook and to focus on the things that you do like about yourself.

The bottom line? Transforming your physique can offer a massive confidence boost. That's because it will impact on the way that other people react to you, it will fill your system with more positive hormones and neurotransmitters to make you feel good about yourself and it will mean you can take care of yourself physically.

So how do you do it? So, let's fix both these aspects, shall we?

The Best Physique

In order to get the kind of physique that will make you feel highly confident, you need to focus on an aesthetic physique. Whether you are a man or a woman, you want a body that you can feel good about and that will make itself known even through clothes.

For guys, that means focusing on the inverted triangle physique. That means wide shoulders, big arms, and a narrow waist. This makes you look physically intimidating and it is a shape that women are naturally inclined to find attractive.

For women, it means developing the hip to waist ratio. This suggests strong genetic material. They should also try to develop a toned physique so that they are proportionate while slim.

In both cases, the best way to accomplish this is with a combination of resistance training and cardiovascular training. And that can even mean combining the two in a manner that is known as concurrent training.

The point is, you shouldn't focus simply on one or the other. Men who only focus on weights will risk looking strong while still carrying a gut. Women who focus only on CV will find they actually don't burn fat as quickly as they would if they combined it with weights. And in fact, women who squat are so well proportioned that it has become a meme!

The style for Women

When it comes to the way you dress there are a few things to consider. This is what 'fashion' is all about. You can't write off the rules of fashion because following fashion demonstrates that you follow social norms and conventions, that you know what is in vogue right now and that you are in touch. Being unfashionable suggests that you are a little clueless or so involved in your own little world that you missed the fact that flares went out of fashion in the 70s.

You don't have to be a slave to fashion, but demonstrating some understanding of what is right now in vogue is highly advisable.

But at the same time, you should also have your own style and you should be willing to take measured risks from time to time.

This is the interplay between fashion and style. Style is the part where you take chances, where you demonstrate your own personality and where you are confident enough to go against the grain. But it all must be done within the rules of fashion. The most important role of your clothes is to make you look awesome. And this means selling your best physical traits in order to ensure you look like a good genetic catch.

Finding your own style is a great way to feel more confident about the clothes you wear. Look to fashion magazines, catalogues and your stylish friends and associates for the inspiration, but then create a look that's entirely your own. Whether you prefer a tailored look or a hippie bohemian style, whatever makes you feel comfortable with yourself is the right choice.

There are times when you'll need to ignore this personal style and wear clothes that are appropriate for a certain occasion. When you're faced with such an event, or even if you have to do it every day for your job, find a way to make the required dress work for you, perhaps by adding your own style with subtle accessories. And if you just can't think of a way to feel comfortable in a tuxedo or the lime green bridesmaid dress your friend selected, draw confidence from the fact that everyone around you feels the same way.

When it comes to clothes, the most important thing is to wear items that make you feel confident and avoid everything else. If you have a shirt that clings to your stomach and makes you feel incredibly fat, then the obvious answer is to not wear that shirt anymore. Too many people would continue to wear the shirt and feel their self-confidence drop every time they put it on. Find pieces that work with your body type and your best natural attributes. If you're not sure how to do it, ask your most stylish friend or family member or find a full-service clothing store.

If you feel like your body type gets in the way of looking your best, maybe you're just not making the best choices. Don't be embarrassed about shopping in the "Women's" department, the "Petite" section or a "Big and Tall" store if that's where you'll find the clothing that fits you best. If you're accustomed to buying your clothes at discount stores, investing in some more expensive but high-quality pieces can result in a better fit because of the better craftsmanship.

Support garments like control-top pantyhose can improve your silhouette and the way you feel about yourself.

Jewelry can add to a polished look. Select pieces that complement and mesh with your chosen style. Don't forget other details as well when you choose accessories. A stylish hat or a fun pair of shoes can bring it all together.

Glasses are another issue when it comes to accessorizing. Some people hate the idea of wearing glasses because they think they look too bookish or it makes them feel old to need reading glasses. Contacts or laser eye surgery may be a suitable option if the idea of wearing glasses is that hateful and detrimental to self-confidence. Alternately, some use their need to wear glasses as an opportunity to show their fashion sense. They choose stylish or trendy frames that complement their faces and improve their confidence in their overall appearance.

Now you're sure to run into people along the way who just want to bring you down. They may scoff at your personal style or your lack of designer clothing or any other detail they can think of to make them feel better about themselves.

Know that this will happen and prepare for it. Whether you want to create snappy comebacks ahead of time or you just want to brace yourself for an insult, being prepared will keep the hateful words from sinking in and affecting the way you feel about your dress. If you're facing these attacks regularly, it may be time to find a new group of friends, remove yourself from the situation, or whatever would lead to a happier you. The saying, "Clothes make the man" may or may not be true, but with the right choices, clothes can make or break your self-confidence.

Physique

As for your body, there is really no space in this book to go through an entire training program!

But first, recognize the importance of investing time and effort into your physique. This is one of the most prominent social signals we put out and one of the most powerful ways to make ourselves feel more confident and successful.

Not only that but being physically superior to someone you're speaking to will infuse you with infinite confidence.

At the end of the day, this is so often what it comes down to. If you are more powerful than the person you're speaking to, then you will be able to beat them in a physical confrontation. Thus, if they don't like what you say and they challenge you, you can put them in their place physically if you have to. And that means you'll have the edge in every conversation. Especially if your physicality communicates this fact.

The basic things to know about getting into this kind of shape:

- Training 3 times per week is generally enough to drastically enhance your size and strength
- Resistance cardio is an incredibly potent method for weight loss and body recomposition – this means performing the cardio exercise while there is a weight of some sort against you
- Diet is every bit as important as exercise. Track your calories and consume more than you burn to increase your size or less than you burn to lose weight.

- Eat more protein to add muscle
- Going to a class or something can help structure your recomposition and make training more fun
- In particular, that means something like a dance class or martial arts. This has the added bonus of making you more functional, meaning that the strength is useable
- For conveying size and power, you should place emphasis on shoulders, chest, and arms. The incline bench press is among the very best exercises you can do.
- For women, the squat or the kettlebell swing is fantastic for developing the most desirable proportions

Chapter 14

Knowing Your Mission

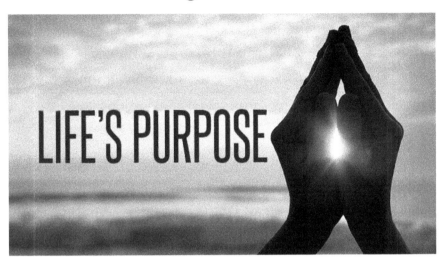

All those tips will help you to massively boost your confidence. But nothing is as powerful as this next tip: know what your mission is. Know what your passion is.

Have something for which you feel truly excited and want to get up every morning for.

Our self-esteem and our confidence are linked to how successful we are and how good we are at things that matter to us. This can mean that our self-esteem is tied up in how we feel we perform in social settings because that's what matters to us.

But now imagine that you're a professional swimmer. Swimming is your passion. So, in social interactions, you're less concerned with what other people think because swimming is what matters to you and you know that you're good at swimming.

Having a 'thing' like this can give you a sense of purpose, of success and of worth. And it can make you socially 'untouchable' in a whole manner of different ways.

And this also means that you are naturally being yourself more and naturally eschewing those social conventions. Because you're following your passion.

Is it any wonder you feel unconfident at work when the work you're doing is something you don't care about and don't feel that you're particularly good at? Imagine if you followed your heart and did something you were truly passionate about: you'd be so much more enthusiastic and confident in your own abilities!

Charisma

And guess what? Being absolutely passionate about something is also something that is known to give people charisma.

Charisma is what happens when we speak with someone who seems to completely enrapture us in what they're saying. We hang off of their every word because they are so magnetic and so compelling.

And it turns out that the people who are most charismatic are the people who gesticulate most, who walk around most and who use their body language the most.

And guess what makes you do this more? Being highly passionate about what you're speaking about. Because when someone talks with passion and fire, their body language becomes naturally congruent with what they're saying. And they become so enthused and so keen for their topic that they can't help but let their body express what they're saying. And people can't help but watch because it is so engaging and because they can pick up on that incredible conviction.

Being in Flow

What's more, is that being highly passionate about something puts us in a state called 'flow'. Flow is kind of like a more positive version of the fight or flight response. This is what happens when we're so focused on what we're doing and when it feels so important to us, that everything else in the world almost seems to just 'fall away'.

The prefrontal cortex shuts down again and this removes that nagging voice. At the same time, our brain is filled with serotonin and anandamide (happiness hormones) along with alertness hormones like dopamine, adrenaline, etc.

In short, you become completely fixated not because you're scared for your life but because you are inspired. And this is the opposite of lacking in confidence. Flow states make conversations flow smoothly, they improve our reactions and they make us magnetic.

So find what you love doing, spend more time doing that and then you'll have a mission. You'll have a purpose. And you'll spend large amounts of inflow and speaking in an animated and engaging way. Confidence will flow naturally out from that.

When you are truly passionate about something you do and you are confident in your ability in that capacity, then you have no need to try and impress people, to overcompensate, etc. Instead, you can be happy in the knowledge that the thing you really care about is going well. That you have reason to be confident.

Now you don't need to try and 'fit in' and there's no reason you can't be kind, generous and sharing with the people you meet in other walks of life.

Conclusion

Now you have the complete picture and hopefully, you've learned a lot about what makes you tick, about where your own anxieties come from and about how you can transform into a more confident, social and happy version of yourself. While they are easy to read about, if you don't take action, the information you've gathered will be meaningless.

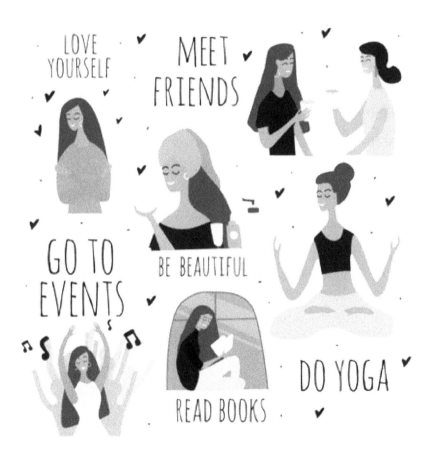

The effort you make in overcoming your limiting beliefs and increasing your confidence will set you apart from everyone else who desires more but has yet to take the necessary steps to move forward.

While you may feel frightened by this action, it is important to remember that all fear that you experience is in your mind. You can overcome it. It just takes a little push of your willpower to get the ball moving.

Take some time to think about which simple confidence hacks you can begin to implement today. It is often far easier to pick one technique and master it before moving on to the next. Confidence, or lack of confidence in your case, doesn't develop overnight, so be patient with the process. Whatever path you choose to take, you are one step closer to reaching your ultimate goal of boosting your self-esteem and building your confidence, so you can finally begin living the life you've always dreamed.